Proton Therapy Destroys Cancer

Revolutionary new technology for <u>80%</u> of ALL cancer types

2020 Edition

Robert Ferré

PROTON THERAPY DESTROYS CANCER
Revolutionary technology for
80% of ALL cancer types

First Print Edition: August 2018
Revised and retitled: January 2020

ISBN: 978-1-940875-82-8 (print)

Library of Congress: (pending)

Published by Labyrinth Enterprises, LLC

www.labyrinth-enterprises.com
San Antonio, Texas

TABLE OF CONTENTS

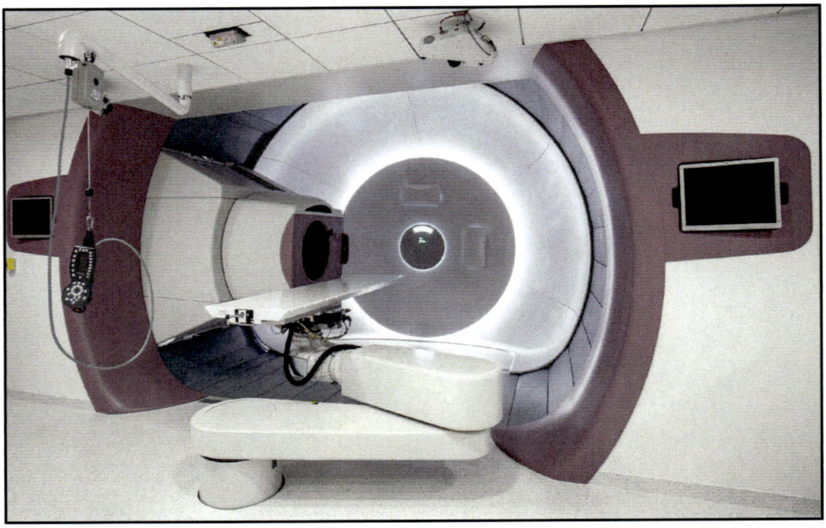

The patient lies on the treatment table. The proton-beaming nozzle adjusts to any angle 360 degrees around the patient. Accuracy is one of the hallmarks of proton therapy, also called proton beam therapy.

NO MEDICAL ADVICE

This book describes proton therapy from my personal point of view as a previous patient treated with this technology. I am NOT giving medical advice. If you think you might want to have proton therapy, contact a proton center and ask for a consultation. Do NOT rely solely on the contents of this book.

Seek a second opinion from a source currently engaged in the application of proton therapy. You may contact me for corrections to this book or to elaborate on my personal opinion, but NOT for medical advice, for which I am unqualified. I do, you will notice, have very strongly held views, which I express freely in these pages. This is not a scientific report filled with footnotes and attributions. Nor have I sought to give critics an equal voice. This is a personal account of the superlative nature of proton therapy. If you disagree with me, feel free to write your own book.

DEDICATION

Ruthie, this book is dedicated to you. You fought breast cancer for six years until taken home at the premature age of 62. If we had known about proton therapy then, you might well have recovered. You will always be in my heart.

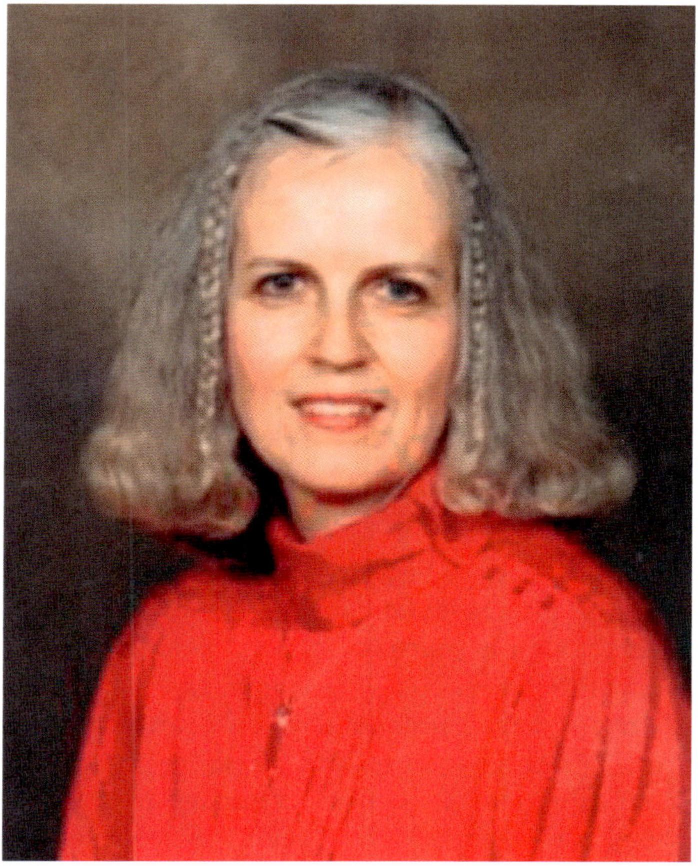

Ruth Hanna

THE BEST TREATMENT YOU NEVER HEARD OF

Proton therapy was developed after World War II by Robert Wilson who had participated in making the atomic bomb. He decided to use his expertise for the benefit of humanity. Over some forty years, proton therapy went through many stages of experimentation. In 1990 the first hospital opened a proton therapy center, in Loma Linda, California. In the subsequent twenty-nine years, thirty-one more centers have opened. Countless people have noticed "Proton Therapy Center" on the front of a building without really knowing what it is.

Proton therapy is a type of radiation that directs streams of charged particles (protons) instead of X-rays. It holds great promise as one of the most effective treatments for cancer. The protons steal electrons from the cancer cells, destabilizing them to the point that they can't reproduce, thereby killing the cancer. Because of the physics involved, proton therapy is extremely accurate, affects very little healthy tissue, and causes few side effects. Best of all, it can be used for 80% of all types of cancer.

Why, then, isn't proton therapy widely known? Why aren't the proton centers besieged by patients? As with the arrival of any new technology, proton therapy has experienced resistance from several sources. First is your family doctor who works long hours and hasn't had time to become familiar with proton therapy. She has always referred her cancer patients for X-rays and continues to do so. To cover her ignorance, she may call proton therapy new, unproven, or experimental. Similarly, radiologists who make their living giving X-ray treatments don't refer their patients for proton therapy, even if it is superior (a fact they are slow to admit). Even within a health system that has a proton therapy center, radiologists fail to send their patients there. They are protecting their own turf. How can they make a living if they send their patients elsewhere?

Added to this list of critics are insurance companies. What they really don't like is how expensive proton therapy is, but the reason they give for not covering it is usually that it is not medically necessary (even if doctors say it is). Recent court cases have awarded substantial judgments against insurance companies that wrongfully denied proton therapy. And finally, the internet is filled with misinformation, often based on old outdated studies that are no longer applicable.

Now, you understand why I, as a proton therapy recipient and advocate, have felt it necessary to write this book. My observations may differ from what your doctor tells you. Shockingly, those people most in need of learning about proton therapy are least likely to find it. In too many cases, they unquestioningly follow the advice of someone who knows nothing about proton therapy or is prejudiced against it.

You, dear reader, are different. You have taken it upon yourself, whether for your own diagnosis or that of a loved one, to research your options. That's exactly what I did when I learned had prostate cancer. Once I had understood all the modalities available to treat my cancer, I chose proton therapy. This book serves as an introduction to the amazing potential and possibilities of proton therapy. It covers the technology and how it is applied, as well as social influences and prospects for the future.

Armed with your new knowledge, you will be in a better position to discuss proton therapy with your doctor to help determine your best treatment plan. If your doctor is not receptive to proton therapy, seek a second opinion, which is standard practice in such critical situations. You may wish to contact a physician at any of the proton therapy centers listed in this book and schedule a consultation. It could save your life and livelihood.

Neither I nor Labyrinth Enterprises LLC shall be liable for any loss or damage allegedly arising from the content of this book. On the other hand, we are proud to take credit for the many people who discover here a revolutionary cancer treatment that will serve them well in their journey to health and wholeness.

1
HOW PROTONS WORK

Protons are particles located in the nucleus of atoms. Their positive magnetic charge is balanced by the negative charge of the electrons that orbit around the atom. Unlike the electrons, protons have mass, which is to say, weight. If I were an electron (175 pounds), my corresponding proton would weigh sixty tons. Tons! Hence, protons behave very differently from, for example, X-rays which have negligible mass.

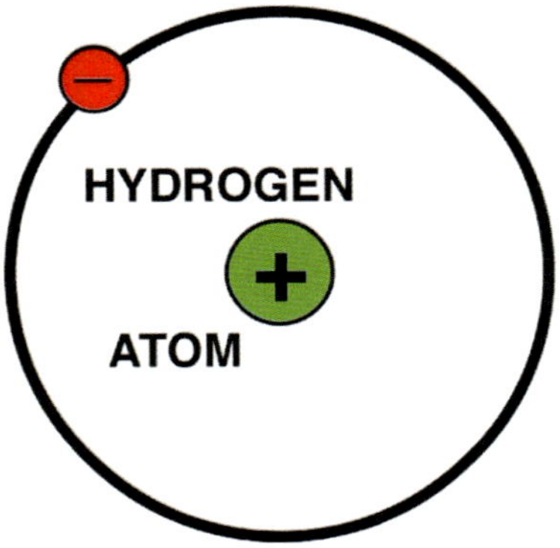

Hydrogen is the best source of protons as it is the most common element in the universe. It has a single electron and a single proton.

Using highly technical equipment (cyclotron, vacuum lines, superconducting magnets), protons are organized into a beam that is classified as a type of radiation. Accordingly, protons are often compared with X-rays—another form of radiation used to treat cancer. There's a vigorous discussion about which is better, X-rays or protons. As both are capable of killing cancer cells they can be called equally effective, but protons:

- Offer greater accuracy
- Are three-dimensional
- Require less radiation
- Produce fewer side effects
- Cause less destruction to healthy tissue

Hence, I believe proton therapy is a technology with a great future and will likely supplant X-rays.

Consider how X-rays work. Because they have so little mass, when X-rays go through the body, many tend to get deflected or to stray. Therefore, to have the full number of X-rays reach the target (a malignant tumor), you must start with a dose as much as 60% higher to make up for the X-rays that are lost. Then, after hitting the target, X-rays keep going until they come out the other side of the body. On both entry and exit, they adversely affect healthy tissue.

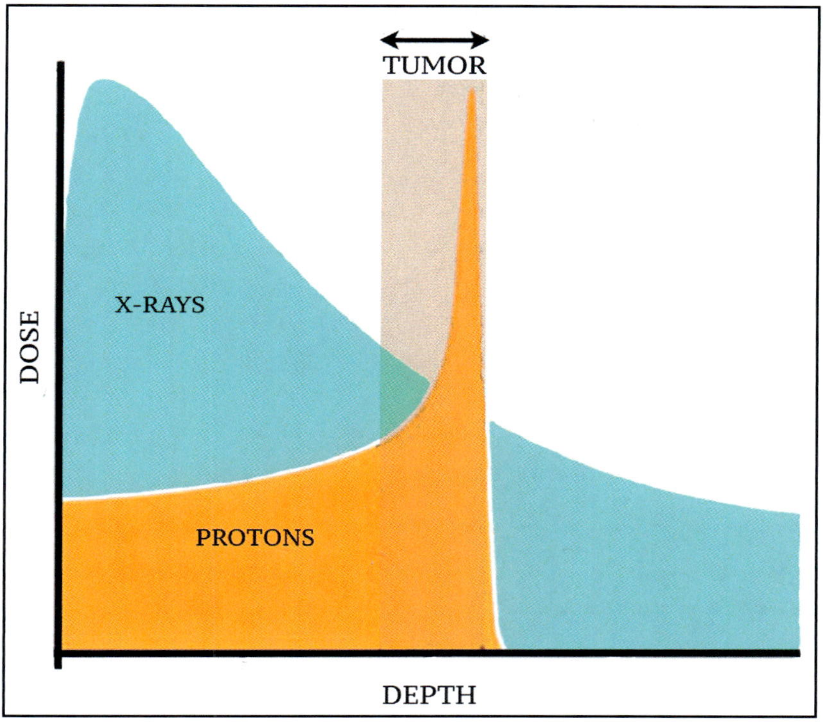

This chart illustrates the difference between X-rays (blue) and protons (orange). With X-rays, the initial dose must be higher. Protons, however, start with a smaller dose, reach a sudden peak of energy and then stop. This is called the Bragg's Peak. It's this phenomenon that allows protons to spare healthy tissue. The energy release takes place within the tumor.

To give better coverage, instead of using a single Bragg's Peak physicists create a series of peaks called the Spread Out Bragg's Peak (SOBP).

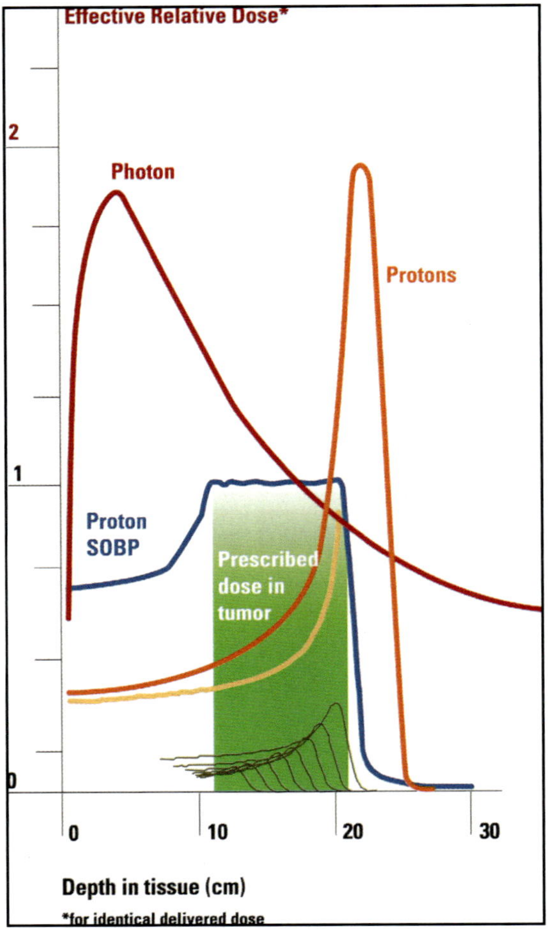

Protons act much differently than X-rays. Having mass, they don't stray. As they enter the body, the protons pick up negatively-charged electrons to stabilize themselves. There is an inverse relationship between speed and energy. As the protons slow down, they release more energy. That's why they enter the body at a lower dose than X-rays. When they slow to a certain speed, they release a burst of energy all at once. This is the Bragg's Peak mentioned above, and the Spread Out Bragg's Peak (SOBP), as shown to the left. They become natural hydrogen again and stop. The point of the energy release can be calculated to happen within the target. This is the unique characteristic of proton therapy that makes it so effective in killing cancer. The protons take their electrons from the cancer cells, which become destabilized and cannot reproduce.

This is the main message of this book, so let me repeat myself. The protons go to their target, release their energy, and stop. There is no exit route as with X-rays. It is amazing to me how science could even figure this out. Thank you Robert Wilson.

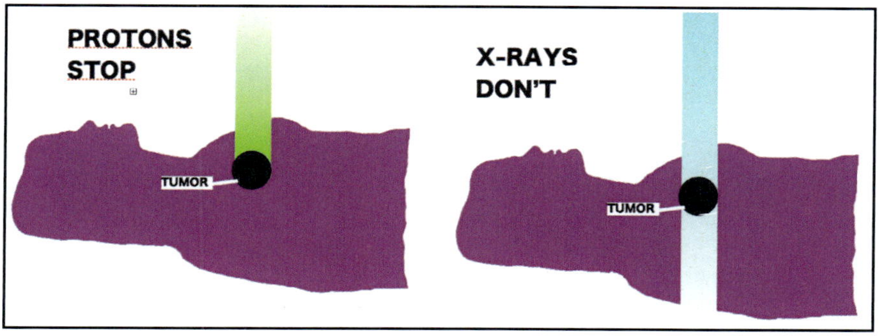

Joke: A proton and an X-ray stop at a bar on the way home from the cyclotron. They'd had a couple of drinks when the bartender came around and asked if they want another round. In slurred speech, the X-ray said, "Sure, let's keep going." But the proton demurs saying, "No thanks. I know when to stop."

Suppose the tumor is shaped like a "U" wrapped around a vital organ. With protons, you can treat half of the "U" from one side and half from the other side without radiating the inside of the "U." With X-rays, the beam goes right across the "U" and radiates the healthy tissue in the middle. It can't be avoided. Because they stop, protons have access to difficult areas where X-rays fear to go.

In the event you are just perusing the beginning pages of this book, here are some quick links where you can find more information. (Snap a photo with your cellphone.)

www.ProtonTherapyBook.com

This site supports my books. It includes most of the color illustrations and photos (with captions) for those who have bought the black-and-white or ebook versions, or no book at all.

www.proton-therapy-centers.com

This site lists operating and planned proton therapy centers in the United States. The same list is at the end of this book.

www.proton-beam-therapy.com

My blog, this site contains newsletters, articles, and links pertaining to proton therapy. Expand your knowledge,

If this book spurs you on to more reading, here is my other book on the subject, specifically for prostate cancer:

Prostate Cancer Conquered with Proton Therapy

With full-color illustrations and photos, this book details my personal experiences as I went through treatment. Although it pertains to prostate cancer, much of the book is relevant to all types of cancer. There is a considerable overlap with material in this book.

These and future books are available on kindle. If you have a black-and-white kindle, you can download the free app to your computer or iPad to enjoy the full color.

Two atoms go into a bar and have a few drinks. The first atom gets a little tipsy and falls off the bar stool.
Second atom: "Are you okay?"
First atom: "No, I don't think so. I think I lost an electron."
Second atom: "That would be terrible. Are you sure?"
First atom: "I'm positive."

Get it? Lost an electron, so he was positive! If these were hydrogen atoms, it would make the first atom that lost its electron a positively charged proton.

2

THE TECHNOLOGY IN DETAIL

Now that we know what protons do, let's look at how they are produced and controlled. Essentially, proton therapy requires a source of protons, an accelerator to ramp up the energy, a selection system to adjust the energy level, a magnet-controlled vacuum line to transport the protons, a delivery system, and a positioning system to adjust the beam, the patient, or both.

An electric charge zaps hydrogen gas to ionize (destabilize) it. Magnets draw off the positively charged protons and inject them into a cyclotron (or synchrotron) where they are accelerated until they reach two-thirds the speed of light. At that speed they would go around the earth five times in one second. One second!

Physicists measure proton energy in electron volts, eV, using MeV to represent a million electron volts. Cyclotrons can energize protons as much as 250 MeV or as low as 70 MeV.

Once at the proper energy level, the protons travel down a beam line within a vacuum (to keep them from contamination from ambient air) except for one place called the degrader. Since all the protons emerge from the cyclotron with the same energy, to vary that energy (and thus the distance the proton beam travels) requires an intervention in the form of a degrader. It looks like a wedge wrapped around a cylinder. Depending on the position of the cylinder, the protons travel through more or less attenuating material.

Exiting the degrader, the protons travel through a vacuum line in which they are shaped and controlled into an organized beam by magnets. Being positively charged, protons naturally repel each other (like the same poles of magnets), trying to spread out. If that happens, the protons get disorganized and bombard the tube, making it radioactive. To prevent this, strong magnets push the protons together in an organized beam (hence, proton *beam* therapy). The quality and consistency of the beam are of the utmost importance. Twenty-four hours a day engineers monitor, test, and calibrate the beam.

PROTON TECHNOLOGY

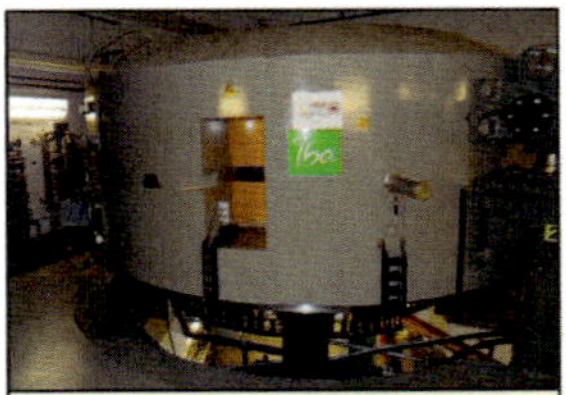

Cyclotron accelerates protons to two-thirds the speed of light

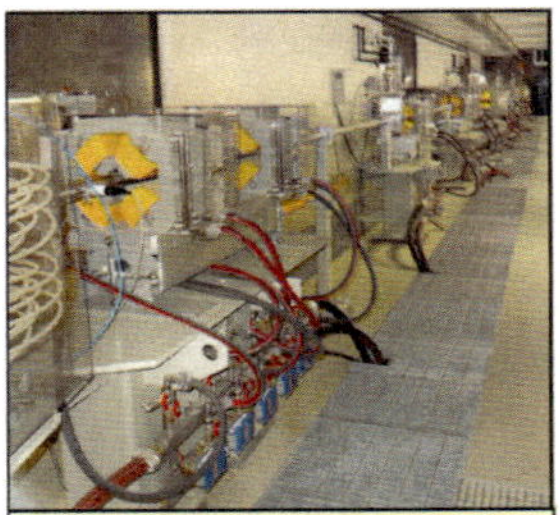

Magnets shape and control protons through beam line

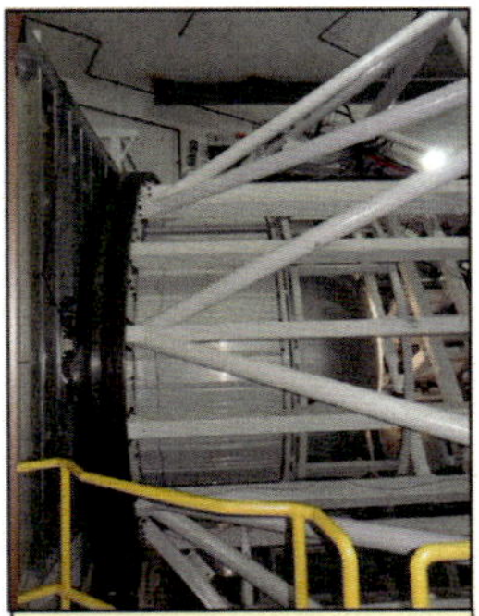

Huge gantry turns the beam a range of 360 degrees

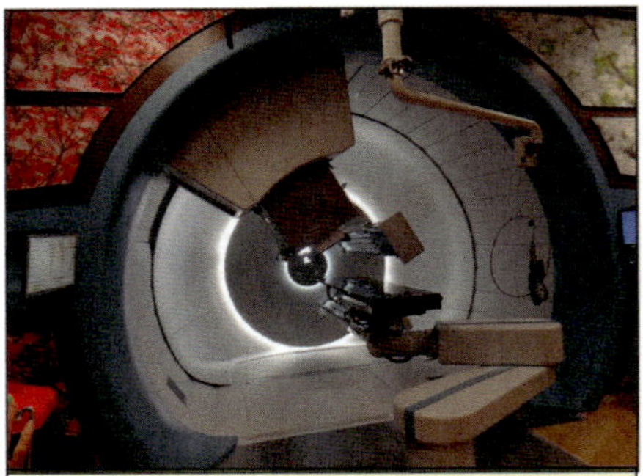

Beam reaches patient on highly adjustable treatment table

To revolve the proton beam 360 degrees around the treatment table looks simple enough. The patient sees a moveable nozzle that rotates with the push of a button. However, behind the wall looms a huge gantry, three stories tall, weighing anywhere from fifty to one hundred and fifty tons, that turns along with the nozzle. Bending the proton beam requires enormously powerful magnets; hence, the weight and size of the gantry. When touring the proton center where I was treated, I was unable to take a complete photo of the gantry because it was so large and I was so close. Hence, in the photo above you see only part of it.

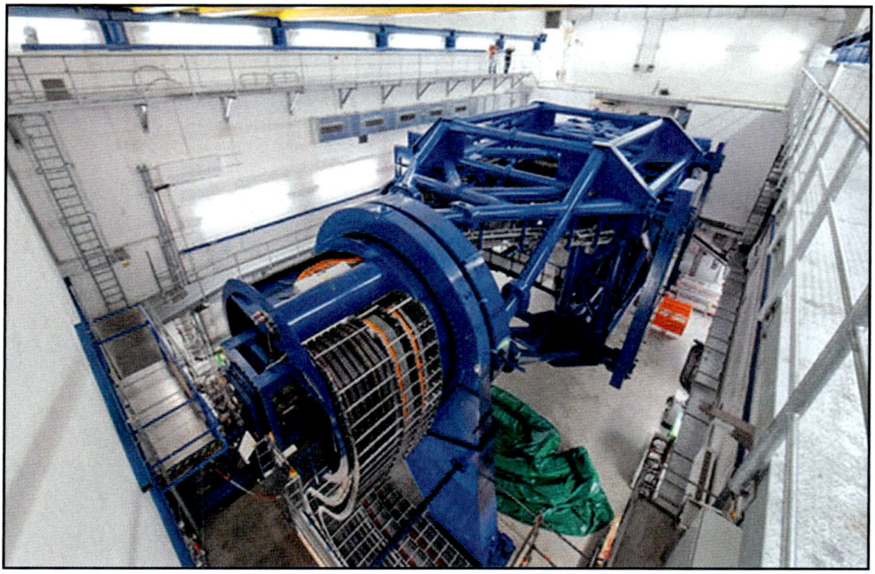

Here is a gantry at Heidelberg University in Germany. Behind the wall on the left is the treatment room. The circular area next to the wall is the tunnel in which the patient lies. When the nozzle moves, the entire gantry turns.

(Used with permission. For information see https://www.heidelberg-university-hospital.com/diseases-treatments/tumor-diseases/proton-therapy-and-carbon-ion-therapy/)

The size and complexity of the equipment, along with the extraordinary requirements for the building that holds it (massive concrete shielding, for example), send the cost for this technology into the stratosphere. Complexity and cost stand as a detriment to widespread development (as does lack of insurance coverage). Your hometown radiologist probably doesn't have a hundred million dollars to spend on proton therapy equipment. Or even thirty million for one treatment room.

Once the gantry turns to its position and the beam reaches the treatment room, it must be directed and controlled to best reach its target. There are two basic ways to do this with protons. The older technology is called double-scattering and produces a rectangular plane that can be shaped by an aperture through which it is directed. For prostate cancer, the patient would have an aperture custom-made to the shape of his prostate. When the plane of scattered protons hits the plate, extraneous ones are screened off while the ones that go forward are the shape of their intended target.

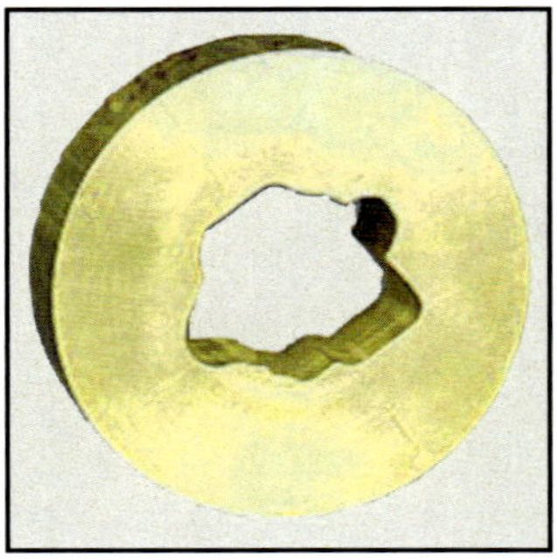

This is an aperture for prostate cancer, made from solid brass. It shapes the beam to protect healthy tissue. It is about five inches across.

The second (newer) method of directing the protons is called pencil beam scanning (PBS). It produces a narrow beam that scans back and forth in layers, laying down little "spots." Each scan can differ, thereby covering irregular shapes.

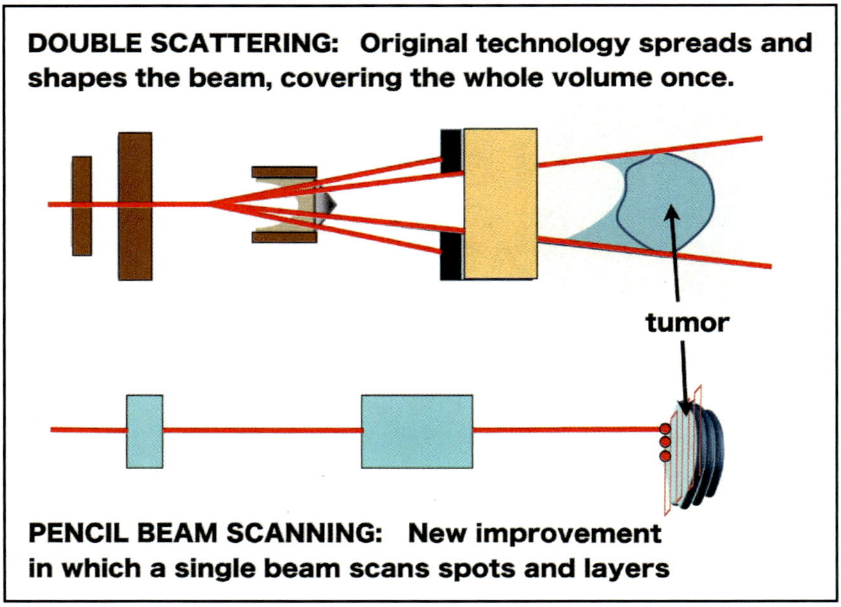

Magnets, modulators, range shifters, apertures, collimators, scatterers, scanners, compensators—all these are used to control and direct the protons to the right place, and that place only.

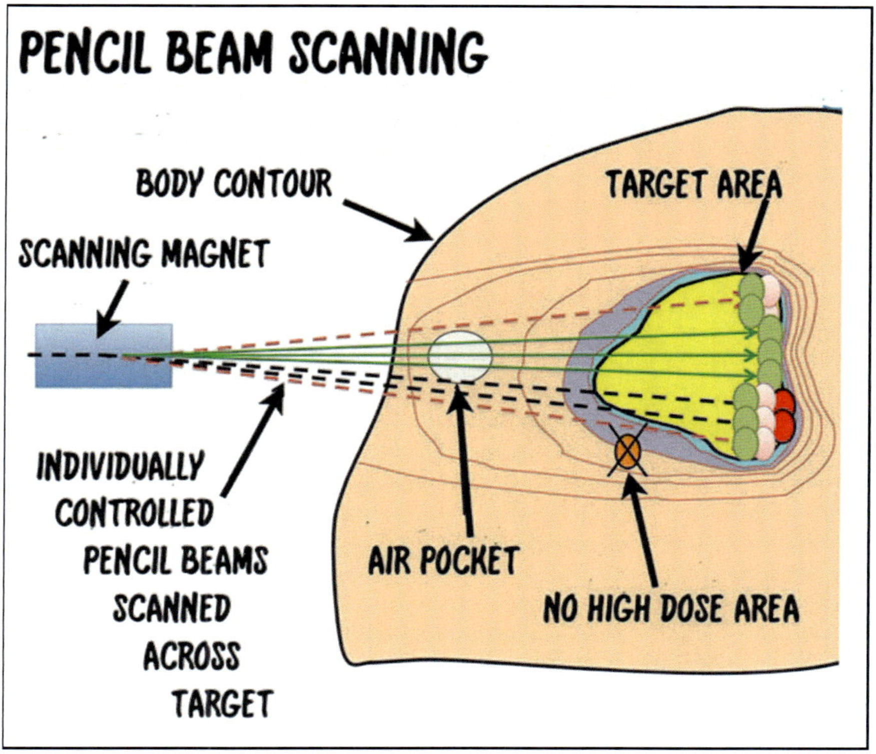

This shows how pencil beam scanning works. If I were seeking a proton center, I would look for one with the newest and most updated technology. Even within PBS, newer versions continue to improve, offering variable beam widths, faster scanning speeds, and other features.

Now that we understand how protons work, we can compare them to X-rays, specifically intensity modulated radiation therapy (IMRT). This modality beams X-rays of lower doses from many directions with the intent of lessening the degree to which it affects healthy tissue. It is this format that radiologists claim gets results similar to proton therapy. However, such claims are based on results of killing the cancer. Yes, both types of radiation do that. But, X-rays do more than that, and more is not better. Let's look at a comparison. The following illustrations are for prostate cancer treatment. Photons are X-rays. (Confusing, no? pHotons and pRotons.)

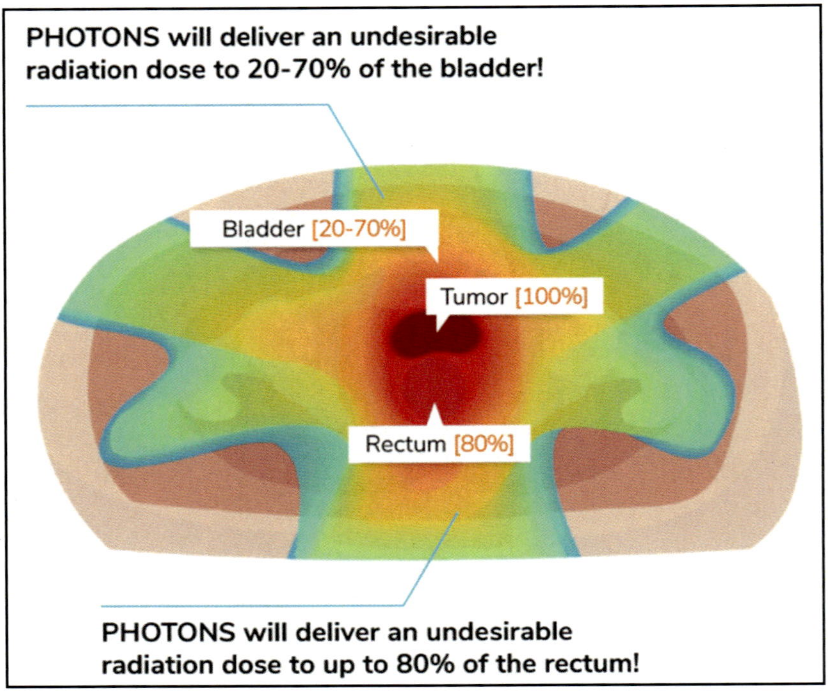

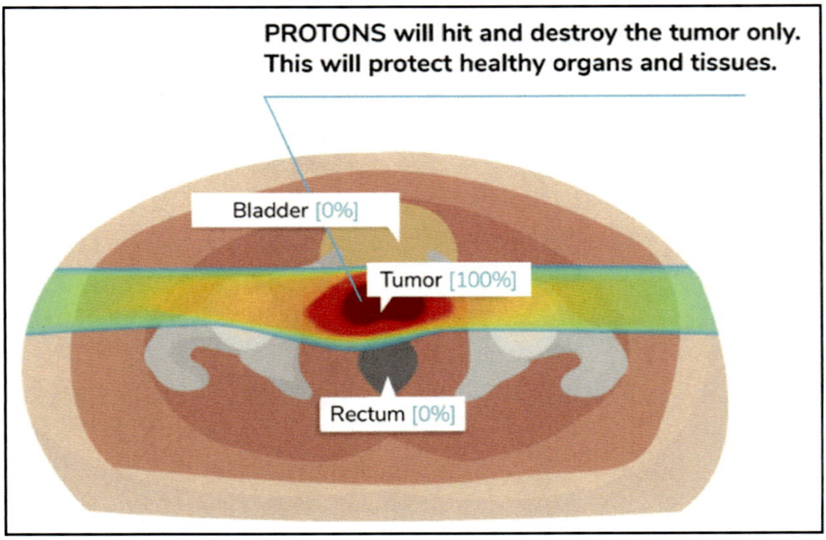

These colorful illustrations were provided by the proton therapy center in Prague. See www.proton-cancer-treatment.com for information. Their graphics really make their point.

Note how protons zero in on the cancer, whereas X-rays overlap the target. Plus, X-rays have a far higher incidence of secondary cancer, caused by the treatment itself. One clever article asked which would you rather have, a smart bomb (protons) or carpet bombing (X-rays).

When the proton beam reaches the patient, additional procedures take place. The first is the use of a range shifter. For my treatment, the range shifter took the form of a removable rectangular screen that slid into the front of the snout (the end of the nozzle), just adjacent to the treatment table. Its purpose is to slow down the beam. With greater resistance, the protons travel a shorter distance. The deeper the protons go into the body the more energy is required. Accuracy involves increasing or decreasing the energy.

As if pencil beam scanning weren't the cat's pajamas, an even more precise technology has been developed called intensity-modulated proton therapy (IMPT) inspired by the X-ray technology called IMRT (the "R" stands for radiation). The proton version, IMPT, lets radiation oncologists adjust the precision, depth, and intensity of a proton beam. The increased accuracy and precision are particularly attractive when treating children with rhabdomyosarcoma, skull base chordoma, and Ewing's sarcoma.

IMPT can vary the size and frequency of the spots, allowing the greatest flexibility. Every beam and spot is calculated in advance. Pencil beam is much less labor intensive and time-consuming than passive double scattered protons. Thereby, more patients can be treated with greater efficiency.

There you have it, the journey of the protons from hydrogen gas, around the cyclotron, through the degrader, down the beam line, rotated by the gantry, into the nozzle, through the range shifter, and into the tumor. But, how do you know how many protons to use? What determines the correct dose? That's the topic of the next chapter. But first, two more illustrations on the next page.

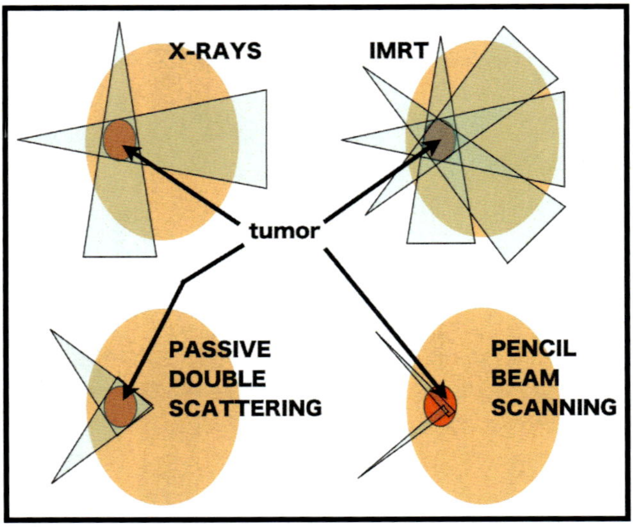

Here, you see the difference between traditional X-rays, intensity modulated radiation therapy, proton double-scattering, and pencil beam scanning. Now that you know what these modalities are, you can see how pencil beam protons are the most accurate and affect the surrounding tissue the least.

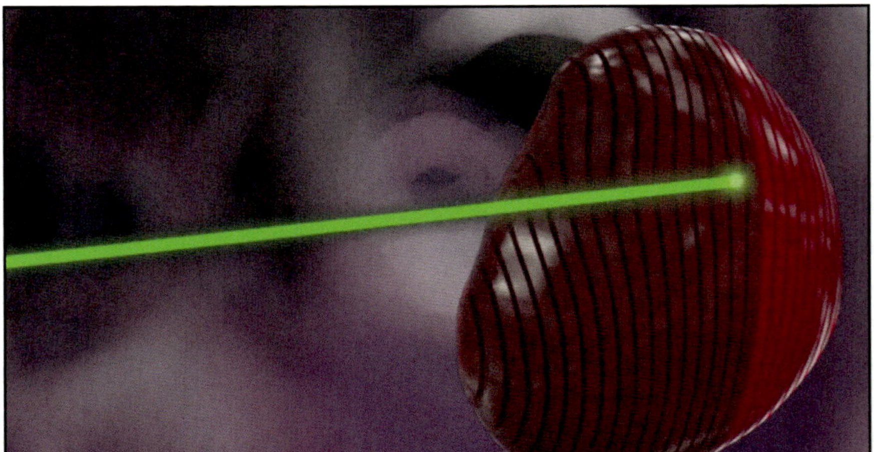

This dramatic illustration of the three-dimensional nature of pencil beam scanning is courtesy of IBA. It shows how the proton spots are laid down in overlapping rows one layer at a time, starting from the most distant.

3

DOSIMETRY DETERMINES THE PROPER DOSE

Dosimetry assures the right number of protons goes to the right place at the right time. In my book about prostate cancer, I include whole chapters on how I was diagnosed and how I decided upon going to Knoxville for treatment. I describe in great detail a typical day of treatment to show the reader the process is very patient friendly and non-threatening.

For medium stage prostate cancer I received thirty-nine treatments, distributed five per week (weekends off). Including a week of preparation, we stayed in Knoxville, Tennessee for two months. My wife Linda and I rented a lovely little furnished cottage, from which we got to know the city and surrounding area. The preparation for each treatment took about ten to fifteen minutes. The actual beaming of the protons took less than two minutes. So, when my treatment was scheduled early in the morning, we had almost the entire day at our disposal. As I experienced no side effects or pain, our activities and lifestyle were not affected. Indeed, we did many more things that we would have done at home.

Famously, some men with prostate cancer play golf every day. We met a woman who was treated for breast cancer at 7:00 a.m. before going to work every day. Others drove themselves as far as ninety miles each day to receive their treatment. Currently there are only thirty-two active proton therapy centers in the United States; unless you live in the area, you must travel there and find lodging. This is one of the detriments for receiving proton therapy, as families or work schedules or other circumstances can make such an extended absence from home difficult. Being retired, we had no problem.

For us, staying in Knoxville was an added benefit. Besides distracting us from the anxiety of cancer treatment, it allowed us to visit friends in North Carolina and Kentucky, and check out Gatlinburg and Pigeon Forge (a month prior to a devastating forest fire that did serious damage).

One key to dosimetry is locating the target accurately. The first step in my case was to have fiducial markers (three little gold beads) permanently imbedded into my prostate.

Next, the doctor injected SpaceOAR hydrogel between my prostate and rectum. The gel is made of two liquids comprised mostly of water; hence the hydro part of Hydrogel.

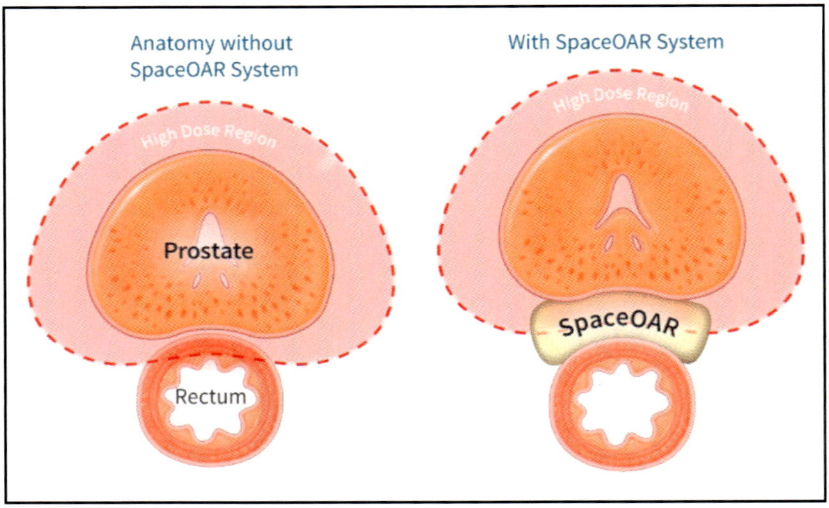

SpaceOAR saves the bacon, if you know what I mean.

The gel pushes the rectum away from the prostate and out of reach of the radiation. After three months it slowly exits the body in the patients' urine, leaving nothing behind. The illustration is courtesy of Augmenix, the manufacturer who bought thirty copies of my book to to use in their training. Hydrogel can be used in other parts of the body as well. For more information on SpaceOAR, see their website (https://www.spaceoar.com/).

The target of proton therapy must remain stable. If the patient moves, then the accuracy could be compromised. When being treated for lung cancer, special procedures are necessary as breathing makes for a moving target. When treating the head or throat, a mesh see-through mask is custom-made for each patient to immobilize the head. For prostate cancer, a leg or body cradle prevents any movement and assures the same position every day.

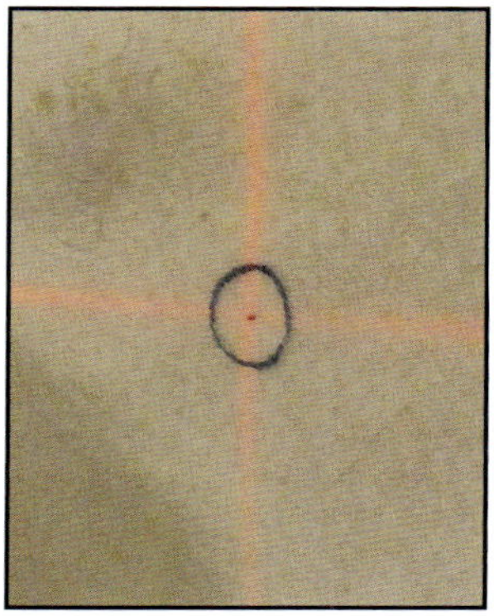

External markers also aid in lining up the proton beam. For a mask, dots or lines can be drawn right on the surface. In my case, I received two little dots, permanent tattoos, one on each thigh. The nozzle was lined up to these dots using laser crosshairs. (See photo. The circle was added with ballpoint pen for the sake of the photo.)

Even with these precautions something can change. The hydrogel may move; the tumor can shrink and change shape; the patient can gain or lose weight. Accordingly, an original baseline must be established against which future treatments can be compared. If need be, the dosimetry can be redone to form a new treatment profile that fits the new circumstances.

Imaging guides the technologists in targeting the protons using equipment such as a cone beam scanner or type of tomography. In my case, they took X-rays each day in which they could see the implanted fiducial markers. On their screen were three images, the initial baseline image, the current one, and a third image that superimposed the first two on top of each other to evaluate any change and confirm accuracy. The images must coincide within a very small tolerance. If not, adjustments and/or reassessments might be necessary. An impressive number of procedures, checks and balances gave a picture of how the treatment was going. All equipment pertaining to my treatment (leg cradle, range shifters, etc.) had bar codes which were scanned during each treatment to verify they were the correct ones for me. If not, a warning would sound. That never happened.

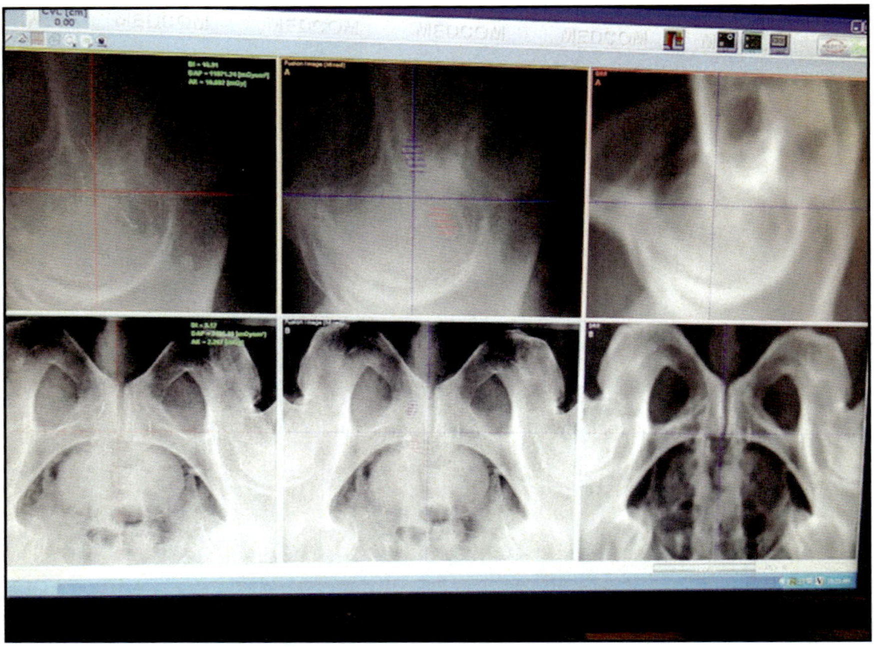

These were my X-rays. I had more than one hundred of them, but they are very low dose. The purpose was to locate my fiducial markers to line up the proton beams accurately.

Daily my oncologist would look at the X-rays to double check the technicians. In the event something was not correct, the computer would sound a warning and prevent the protons from being delivered. That never happened to me.

All these procedures, fiducial markers, scans, baselines, X-rays, bar codes, constant checking by engineers and physicists, and robust dosimetry are part of what is known as Quality Assurance (QA). Proton centers place great importance on proper QA. Even the quality of the proton beam itself is checked during each treatment. At the treatment end of the beam line the protons pass through three consecutive ion chambers that measure the calibration. One time, there was about a two-minute delay while I was on the table. I asked what had happened. The tech said the beam had gone out of calibration. Elsewhere, in a control room, engineers made a quick adjustment and everything then proceeded according to plan.

None of this can be seen by the naked eye. Therefore, it takes constant monitoring by special equipment to assure that the protons are being properly directed. One cyclotron can typically serve three to five treatment rooms. Once the patient is aligned, a ready signal is given. When the proton beam becomes available, it is switched to that room. The wait can be very short or take several minutes. Then, the beam is switched to the next room.

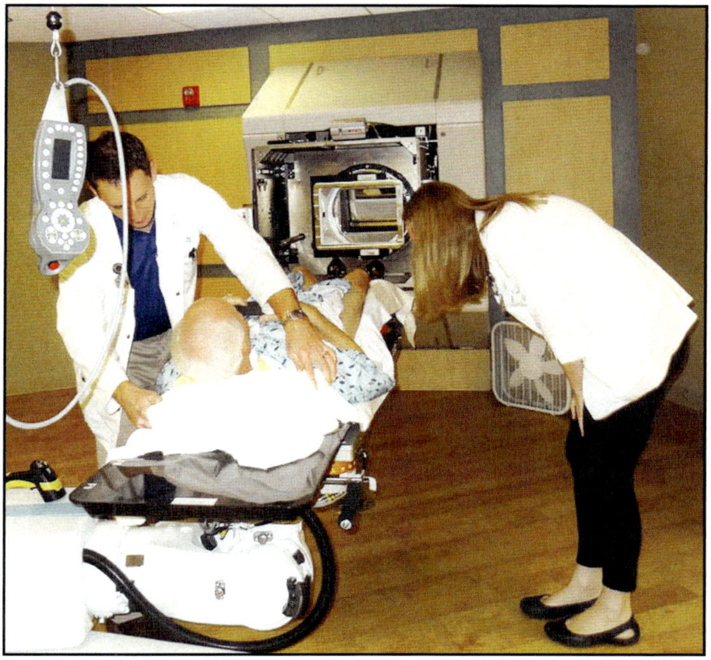

Here, I am on the treatment table. The protons come through the nozzle, visible behind me after the table is turned and lined up using X-rays and laser crosshairs on my tattoos.

Given this description, you can see why proton therapy is expensive. The cost of the building and equipment plus the large staff and skill requirements explains why proton therapy costs more than X-rays. Profitability depends on the number of patients treated. While I never felt rushed, I could tell that the procedures were designed to rotate patients in and out efficiently. While one patient is being treated, the next one is in a dressing room, putting on a hospital gown. As soon as one patient leaves the treatment room the next one arrives with just enough time between for the techs to change cradles, range shifters, computer files and other details. Every day when I arrived they would ask me my birth date and check it with the file on the screen. Once I was in position, the techs sent the proper settings to the degrader and initiated the scan pattern articulated specifically for me. Despite the high technology, in the end, humans must perform with precision. Numerous checks and balances assure that all standards are met.

I got to know members of the staff, the technicians, and many patients. In other accounts I have read about receiving proton therapy, the social component was very important. Some new-found friendships last a lifetime. I'll have to admit to being a bit of a curmudgeon. Linda and I would often sit at a table at one end of the waiting room, keeping to ourselves. I guess each person has his or her own style.

At the beginning, after the setup, the examinations, the scans, the markers, the tattoos, it then took the physicist several days to calculate the exact treatment dose and delivery method. I considered this part so critical to my understanding that I spent several hours with the physicist as he explained exactly what he did for my specific case.

Special software aids in the process. Provision chose Ray Station, designed by a very progressive company located in Stockholm, Sweden. Using scans taken during setup, the physicist manually traced my various internal organs on the screen. His training and experience resulted in considerable expertise in doing this. Once the organs are traced (using different colors for each organ), the image can be moved and rotated to any angle. He showed me a side view, and then a front view and a top view. The computer calculates exactly the right direction from which the protons should be scanned. The software tests various "what if" scenarios to find the best one.

In my case, treatment was directed from each side through the femur heads (top of the major bone in the legs). A gantry wasn't necessary, so I was in a room with a fixed beam. The nozzle just came out of the wall, instead of being mounted on the dramatic circulating device. A study at Mass General Hospital in Boston concluded that 67% of cancers can be treated from a fixed (or slightly adjustable) beam. Eliminating the gantry would drastically reduce the building cost.

Pencil beam scanning, as earlier described, covers the target in rows and layers of tiny overlapping spots. During my treatment, I could hear the movement of the scanning magnets directing each layer of protons, followed by three or four seconds of silence. For thirteen treatments I had sixteen layers comprising 1,962 spots. Then, when the lymph nodes and seminal vesicles were added the plan became thirty-two layers totaling 5,276 spots. One article I read said that PBS can lay down 400 spots per second. That means my beam would take thirteen seconds. During the planning stage, the dosimetrists assembled a twenty-two page document mapping out every layer and every spot for me.

Treatment Site	Start	End	Dose CGE	Fractions	Fields	Tech	Elapsed days
Prostate	9/8/16	9/29/16	32	16	Lat opposed	PBS	21
Prostate/SV/LNs	9/30/16	11/1/16	46	23	Lat opposed	PBS	32
Cumulative Total			78	39			54

Above is a summary I received about my dosimetry plan.

A fraction is a single treatment. The accumulated dose amount of 78 for my treatment refers to a measurement called a Gray (Gy), which represents the absorption of one joule of radiation energy per kilogram of matter. (Don't worry, I don't understand it either.) My dose chart is far from universal. Different proton centers use different approaches. For example, you could have a shorter number of fractions with a higher dose. Or, a lower dose overall.

The proton center in Prague treats prostate cancer in three ways: The first uses five fractions, one administered every other day at 7.25 Gy per fraction (more than three times my dose of 2.0 Gy), used for early stage and low risk cases. Two days between give a little more time for healthy tissue to recover. I believe the Mayo clinic may offer a five fraction plan.

The second plan in Prague calls for nineteen fractions, for people who previously had surgery (the failure of which is apparently a common occurrence!). The third modality applies twenty-one fractions at 3 Gy per fraction. Twenty-one fractions = 63 Gy vs. my thirty-nine fractions = 78 Gy.

The proton therapy center in San Diego treats prostate cancer by spreading a total dose of 90 Gy over five and one-half weeks. The intent remains the same, to kill the cancer and spare the healthy tissue. When it comes to healthy tissue, more radiation is not better. But for killing cancer, higher doses have higher success rates. So, a delicate balance must be achieved.

The chapter on future developments (see p. 92) describes an experimental program using a single large treatment for less than one second. Period. Finished. Surprisingly, it doesn't affect the healthy tissue as much as one would expect.

Now that you have some understanding of the technology and the dosimetry, let's go into more detail about how protons treat a variety of cancers. Prostate cancer has been my focus in describing the workings of proton therapy. Please note that similar techniques and quality assurance exist for all types of cancer listed in the next chapter.

4

TYPES OF CANCERS TREATED WITH PROTON THERAPY

Improvements in proton therapy have greatly increased how many cancers it can treat. The development of pencil beam scanning has especially allowed proton therapy to become a major player. To qualify for proton therapy, the cancer must be locatable. Leukemia, for example, is a systemic cancer without a specific location and would not be a candidate for proton therapy.

Unlike X-rays, the spots of pencil beam scanning can be very specific. Picture a jar filled with red and white marbles mixed together. Pencil beam scanning could treat all the red marbles while largely sparing the white marbles (or vice versa) whereas X-rays would radiate the entire jar.

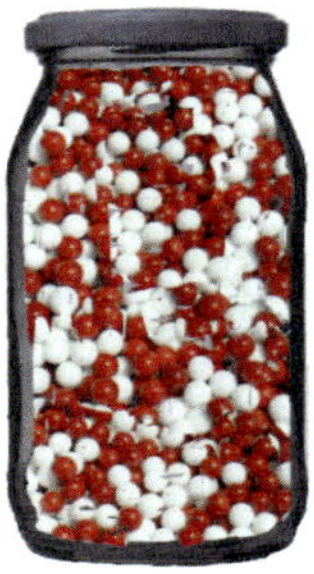

Here are some of the cancers that can be treated with protons. Sometimes, we compare protons and X-rays (photons).

Base of Skull

Acoustic neuromas are benign tumors that press on a cranial nerve often causing hearing loss. As with other sensitive areas, protons do less damage than X-rays and are more effective. Chordomas and chondrosarcomas are tumors of the brain stem, spinal cord, and central nervous system tissue. Proton therapy here spares injury to the brain and spinal cord. Meningiomas are slow-growing tumors in the linings of the brain and spinal cord. These, too, are often benign but they can be difficult to remove because of their location. The proton center in Loma Linda, California, states: “Proton radiation therapy is used for meningiomas to deliver a high dose of radiation in a few treatments. Long-term results show that proton therapy for benign meningiomas yields excellent results with minimal side effects."

Dr. Anita Mahajan, medical director at MD Anderson Proton Therapy Center in Houston, Texas treated a teenage girl with a skull base chordoma. She says this. "The location of her tumor, nestled between the brain stem and spinal cord, was a deciding factor in using IMPT." (IMPT stands for Intensity Modified Proton Therapy, an advanced form of pencil beam scanning.)

Brain Tumors

The superiority of protons for brain tumors has long been acknowledged. Side effects such as nausea and fatigue are greatly reduced.

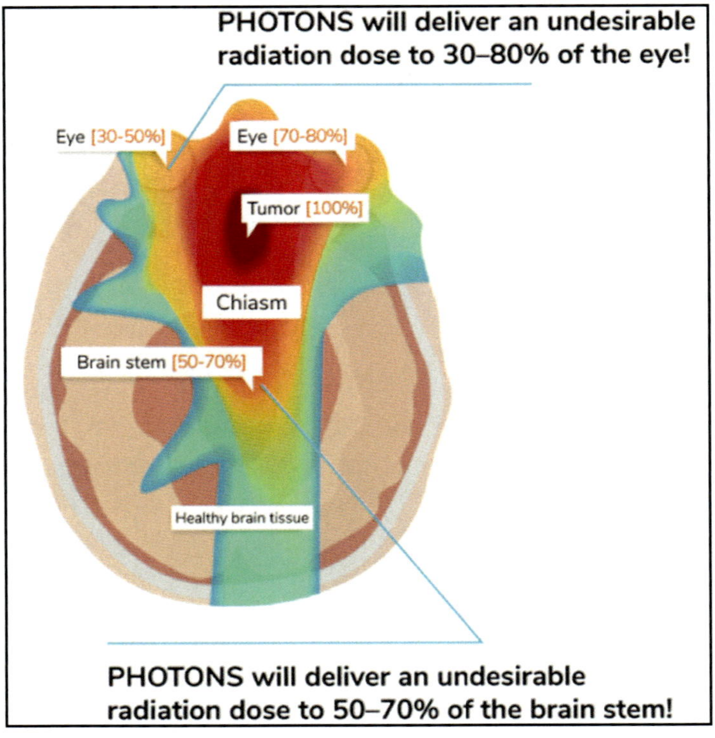

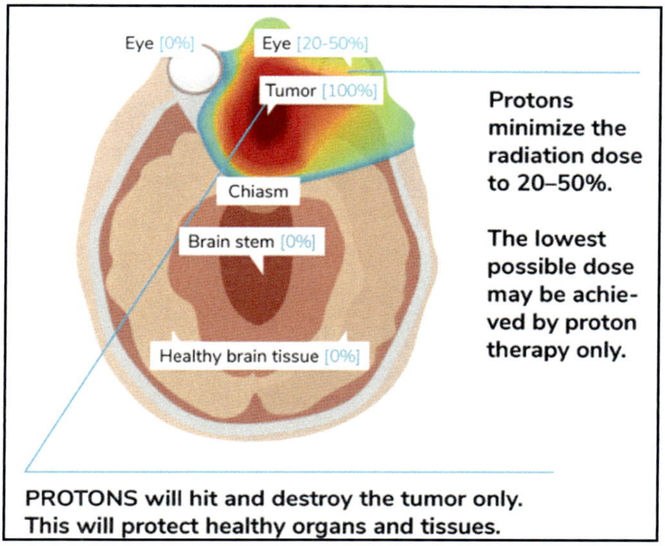

These colorful illustrations compare photons (X-rays) and protons. They were provided by the proton therapy center in Prague, The Czech Republic. See www.proton-cancer-treatment.com for more information.

The Oklahoma Proton Therapy Center lists these as among the types of brain tumors best suited for proton therapy.

Low-grade glioma
Recurrent glioma
Meningioma
Pituitary adenoma
Craniopharyngioma

Protons help protect the eyes, as some treatments leave the patient blind. I can think of few things more scary than a brain tumor. I'd be relieved that proton therapy was possible. At the end of the book is a dramatic story of a family that fled England so their child could get proton therapy for his brain tumor. The went through many hardships, but in the end, he was treated. Instead of becoming a vegetable, he is now a rambunctious young man[53] free of cancer.

Breast Cancer

Treating breast cancer with X-rays can cause physical damage to the lungs and heart. Because protons stop at the tumor, they offer little threat to other organs. When the heart is exposed to X-rays, the resulting heart disease is directly proportional to the dose of radiation received. Repercussions can continue for twenty years. Twenty years! That's definitely a reason to minimize exposure, which is what protons do best.

At the 2017 Particle Therapy Cooperative Group - North America (PTCOG-NA) conference, several significant clinical papers were presented to further support the benefits of proton therapy as a treatment. Here is a summary of one of them.

Initial findings from a multi-institutional study sponsored by the Proton Collaborative Group demonstrated that short-course proton therapy to the partial breast is a safe and effective treatment for select patients with early stage breast cancer. Side effects of treatment were minimal, with no serious treatment-related adverse events reported. Good or excellent breast cosmesis was attained for all patients. There have been no local or distant disease recurrences to date. This study confirms that partial breast irradiation with short-course proton therapy is well tolerated and provides excellent early cancer control.
(see http://www.protonintl.com/index.php/news-posts/napt-calls-attention-to-promising-clinical-trial-results-presented-at-particle-therapy-cooperative-group-meeting-in-chicago)

A study by MD Anderson Cancer Center in Houston revealed that proton therapy is a cost-effective treatment for early-stage breast cancer, compared to other therapies. The study found that the cost of proton therapy when used for accelerated partial breast irradiation (to decrease overall treatment time and toxicity) was estimated at $13,833. Intensity-modulated radiation therapy for whole breast irradiation was $19,599.

For more information, see https://www.mdanderson.org/patients-family/diagnosis-treatment/care-centers-clinics/proton-therapy-center.html.

PHOTONS will deliver an undesirable radiation dose to 12–20 % of the heart!

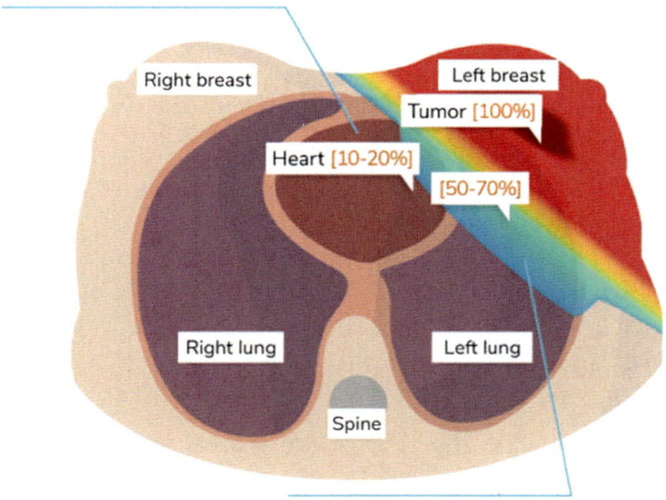

PHOTONS will deliver an undesirable radiation dose to 50–70% of the lung!

PROTONS will hit and destroy the tumor only. This will protect healthy organs and tissues.

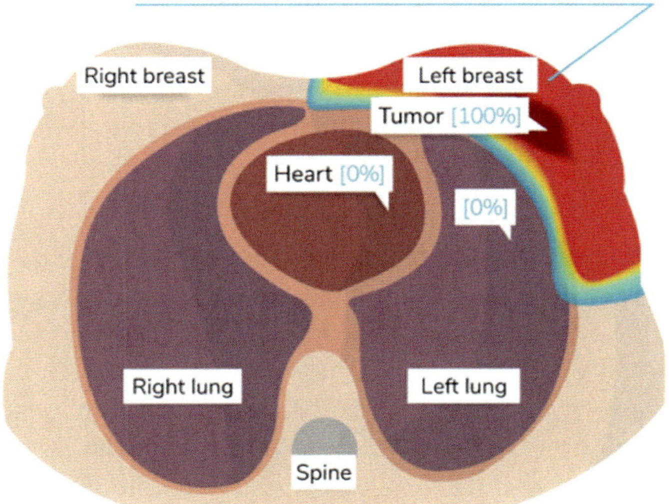

The University of Florida Proton Therapy Center did a five-year study that showed how protons were superior to X-rays for breast cancer. Here is the reference:

Bradley JA, Dagan R, Ho MW, Rutenberg M, Morris CG, Li Z, Mendenhall NP. Initial Report of a Prospective Dosimetric and Clinical Feasibility Trial Demonstrates the Potential of Protons to Increase the Therapeutic Ratio in Breast Cancer Compared With Photons. Int J Radiat Oncol Biol Phys. 2016 May; Vol. 95(1):411-21

Esophageal Cancer

Here is another summary from PTCOG-NA.

Physicians from the MD Anderson Cancer Center, the Mayo Clinic, and the University of Maryland evaluated the impact of different radiation treatments on outcomes for elderly esophageal cancer patients treated with chemotherapy and radiation therapy followed by surgery. The radiation therapy treatments evaluated in the study were 3-D conformal radiation therapy, Intensity Modulated Radiation Therapy (IMRT), and proton therapy. Proton therapy enables physicians to minimize the dose of radiation to the heart and lungs while targeting esophageal cancer. The study results reflected that patients treated with proton therapy had fewer postoperative heart and lung complications such as acute respiratory distress syndrome (ARDS) and heart attacks, shorter hospital stays, and reduced risk of postoperative death than patients treated with other types of radiation.
(See website: ptcog.ch)

Older patients with esophageal cancer not only experience more post-treatment heart and lung problems than younger patients, but they are also at a higher risk for death after receiving a combination of preoperative radiation therapy and chemotherapy. They say proton beam therapy in place of traditional radiation therapy in the preoperative setting has yet to be fully understood. Addressing that question in the above study, researchers assessed outcomes by each type of radiation treatment. Results of the study showed that older patients treated with proton beam therapy benefited from improved outcomes and lower toxicities than the patients treated with either of the other radiation methods. Critics of proton therapy keep demanding comparative studies. Well, here is one, and the determination is unmistakable.

The other issue is recurrence of the cancer. The MD Anderson Clinic in Houston calculated for esophageal cancer, X-rays have a whopping 96% additional cancer risk. That's enough to send anyone to the proton therapy center.

Gastrointestinal (GIT)

Sometimes X-rays or surgery can't reach cancer located in sensitive places because they would damage surrounding organs. Here's what the proton center at MD Anderson in Houston has to say.

By using proton therapy to treat gastrointestinal (GI) cancers, a higher dose of radiation is able to be delivered directly to where it needs to be — to the cancerous cells — while sparing healthy tissues and critical areas of the body such as the liver, kidneys, small bowel and stomach. When treating GI tumors, treatment will often be a combination of surgery, chemotherapy and radiation therapy.

Gastrointestinal cancers we treat with proton therapy are:

Anal cancer
Bile duct cancer
Esophageal cancer
Gastric cancer
Metastatic tumors
Pancreatic cancer
Primary liver cancer
Rectal cancer

On the next page are more of the colorful illustrations from the proton center in Prague. Again, these illustrations don't equivocate. They certainly make their point.

PHOTONS will deliver an undesirable radiation dose to 50–70% of the liver!

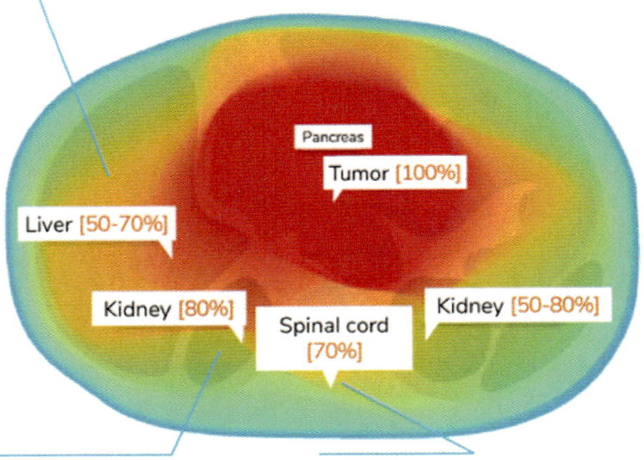

PHOTONS will deliver an undesirable radiation dose to 50–80% of the kidneys!

PHOTONS will deliver an undesirable radiation dose to up to 70% of the spinal cord!

PROTONS will hit and destroy only the tumor. This will protect healthy organs and tissues.

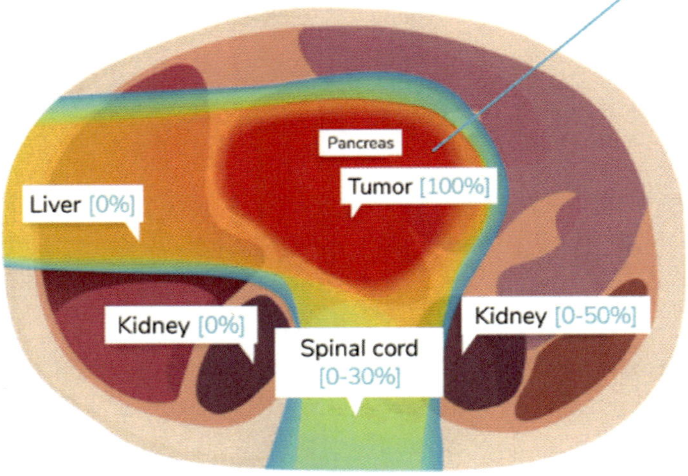

While protons are well recognized for treating some cancers, others are less obvious, as illustrated in the graph below.

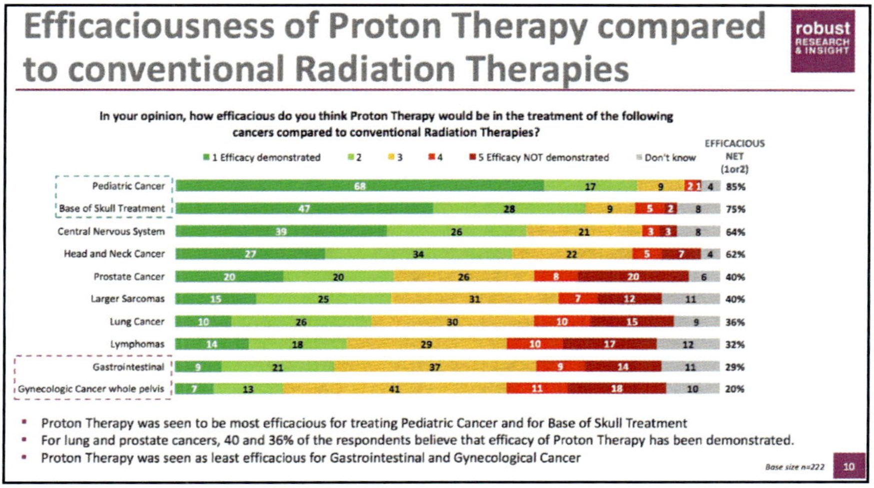

Gastrointestinal cancer is one of the least recognized as being effectively treated with proton therapy. I think over time this will change. The above graph comes from a survey of 222 proton workers conducted by IBA, the leading manufacturer of proton equipment. On their website (www.iba-worldwide.com) they have other white papers and surveys.

Head and Neck

All treatments damage the many sensitive organs in the head and neck area, such as salivary glands, eyes, and optic nerves. It's just a question of how much. With protons, such organs are largely spared, as are side effects such as dry mouth, hearing loss, and blindness. Some critics dismiss the importance of side effects, but I think patients feel differently.

A feeding tube is less frequently required with protons. In Knoxville, I met several fellow patients being treated for head and neck cancers. In one case, the skin showed a large area of radiation burn (like sunburn) and the patient was having difficulty talking and eating. If that was his experience with protons, I can't imagine how much worse it would have been with other modalities. A study by MD Anderson in Houston made the following conclusion comparing IMRT (X-rays) and IMPT (protons).

IMRT is the current standard of treatment for head-and-neck cancer because of its ability to tightly conform the dose to target volume, sparing normal structures such as the parotid glands. IMPT further refines treatment by avoiding high doses of radiation to normal tissue structures. Because of this, neurocognitive function, vision, swallowing, hearing, taste and speech can be better preserved.

(For more information see: https://www.mdanderson.org/patients-family/diagnosis-treatment/care-centers-clinics/proton-therapy-center.html)

The report gives a nod to X-rays but says protons do a better job of preserving some very vital functions.

In the retirement center where I live, one of the staff members twice had a type of throat cancer. The first time she was treated with X-rays. She was seriously burnt and couldn't eat or swallow. She missed two months of work. A year later the cancer returned on the other side. This time she received proton therapy. She had far fewer side effects and returned to work in two weeks. Hearing her description, one cannot fail to be convinced of how superior proton therapy was. Sadly, she had requested proton therapy the first time, but her doctor insisted on X-rays, thereby resulting in additional pain and suffering. Such a circumstance is not unusual.

I feel bad reporting that we can't always believe our doctors. I don't mean to demean the entire profession, yet I have seen numerous cases in which the doctor's interests were put ahead of the patient's. If your doctor had been progressive and recommended proton therapy, you wouldn't probably be reading this book. I feel impelled to encourage people to get a second opinion if their doctor is negative about proton therapy.

Hodgkin's Lymphoma

Hodgkin's lymphoma is a cancer of the immune system. Located in the lymph nodes, it is most often found in children and young adults and compromises the body's ability to fight infection. It's most often diagnosed in those between the ages of 15 and 35 and most often affects those with a family history of lymphoma. Because lymphatic tissue is in many parts of the body, Hodgkin's lymphoma can begin almost anywhere.

Proton therapy is effective for cancer of the lymph nodes because the treated areas don't need to be contiguous. Here's what MD Anderson in Houston says about their treatment of this cancer.

Traditionally, lymphoma is treated with chemotherapy followed by radiation therapy. But, because many lymphomas occur in the chest near critical structures such as the heart, lungs or esophagus, it can be difficult to get the high doses of radiation needed to the tumor without causing damage to those sensitive areas. With proton therapy, our specialized team of cancer experts are able to create a treatment plan that precisely targets even the most difficult to reach lymphoma tumors while minimizing the damage to healthy tissues and vital organs.

Proton therapy is especially valuable in treating patients with lymphoma whose tumors are in the chest or involve the anterior mediastinum, as well as those whose tumors that have proven to be resistant to chemotherapy. For patients with chemotherapy-resistant tumors that require targeted high doses of radiation, proton therapy may be the only hope for curative treatment.

With proton therapy for lymphoma, treatments typically take about 15 to 30 minutes each day and are delivered five days a week for approximately four to seven weeks. The course of treatment and length of time per treatment each day vary based on each patient's individual case. Most patients tolerate the treatments extremely well and are able to continue to work and exercise during their treatment course and immediately after treatment is complete.

(For more information see: https://www.mdanderson.org/patients-family/diagnosis-treatment/care-centers-clinics/proton-therapy-center.html)

While I was being treated for prostate cancer, my dosimetrist showed me how proton therapy "really shines" when it comes to treating the lymph nodes near the prostate. They form a "U" shape (see drawing on p. 57). Proton therapy can treat the lymph nodes from each side, not affecting the organs in the middle of the U. X-rays would go all the way across, hitting everything.

The next illustrations show how X-rays (photons) may deliver strong doses to the heart, lungs, and spinal chord, ranging from 20% to 90%. Proton therapy, in contrast, is shown as having zero effect on these organs. I believe these figures are for illustrative purposes only. There are surely cases in which proton therapy affects some surrounding organs, albeit to a small degree. However, when considering the big picture, protons spare most of the surrounding sensitive organs. Making that point is the purpose of this book.

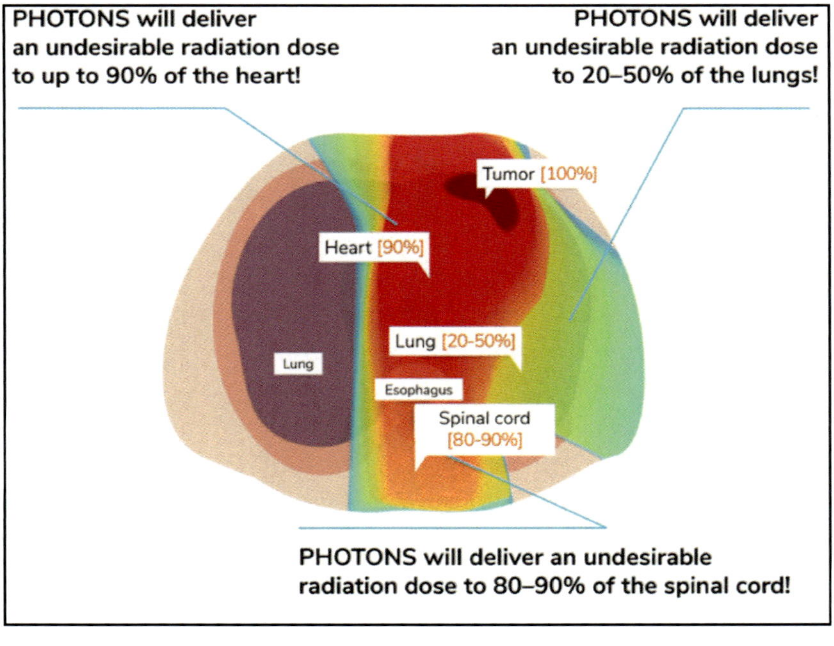

Photons are shown to hit a considerable percentage of organs at risk. There are techniques in which exposure can be reduced, but nothing can make X-rays stop the way protons can.

PROTONS will hit and destroy the tumor only.
This will protect healthy organs and tissues.

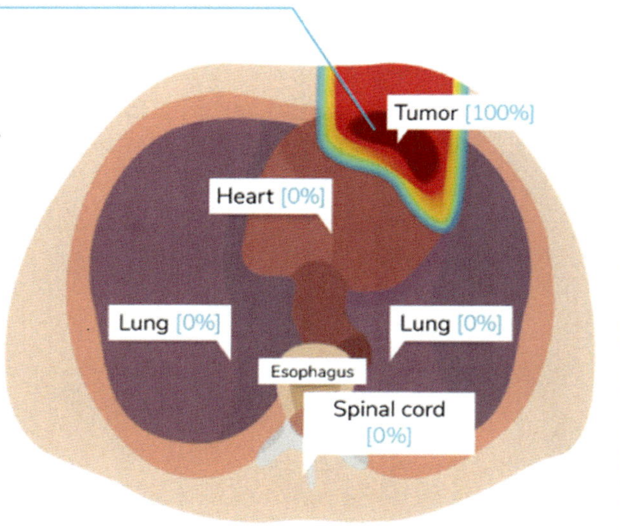

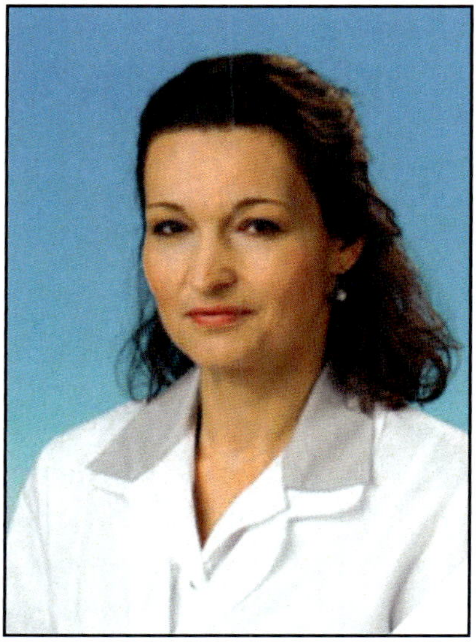

"Proton therapy for the treatment of lymphomas enables the application of a sufficient and effective dose to the tumour while sparing healthy organs such as spinal cord, lung, heart, and mammary glands from the radiation. Proton radiotherapy offers young patients who are mainly affected by this disease the chance of a healthy future. It should always be considered in patients requiring mediastinal radiotherapy or repeated irradiation."

Dr. Katerina Dedeckova, radiation oncologist, proton therapy center in Prague, the Czech Republic.

The mediastinum is the part of the chest that lies between the sternum and the spinal column, between the lungs. This area contains the heart, large blood vessels, trachea, thymus gland, esophagus, and connective tissues. Mediastinal recurrence remains the most common cause of failure in patients with mediastinal T-cell lymphoblastic lymphoma (LBL). In looking up this definition, I found the following statement:

Breast cancer, lung cancer, thyroid cancer, sarcomas, and skin cancer/melanoma are the most common forms. Secondary cancer is a significant cause of death of patients cured for Hodgkin's lymphoma by radiation therapy.

"Significant cause of death!" I wouldn't call death a side effect nor is secondary cancer a cure. Yes, the original cancer was eliminated, but at a very considerable risk of future recurrence. Hence, the need for proton therapy. When I see data like this, it bugs me when critics say there is no difference in the effectiveness of X-rays and protons. Would life or death be considered a significant difference?

Liver Cancer (hepatocellular carcinoma, HCC)

Since blood from all parts of the body must pass through the liver for filtration, cancer cells from other organs and tissues that reach the liver can lodge and grow into secondary tumors.

"We liken the liver to the body's Grand Central Station because all tumor cells circulate through it which is why cancer recurrence is most likely to happen there," said Gary Yang, M.D., professor of radiation medicine at Loma Linda University Medical Center. Dr. Yang is principal investigator of "Stereotactic Body Proton Therapy for Liver Metastases," a study exploring a better way to manage the condition while sparing harmful effects to the liver. Non-invasive proton therapy is given in higher doses than have previously been used with conventional X-ray therapy. In such a case, more is better. Higher doses have more success in killing the cancer.

“Typically invasive open surgery and chemotherapy have been the two main options for controlling liver metastases; but due to patients’ immune systems being compromised or because they are weak, aged, and/or frail, many cannot withstand open surgery,” says Dr. Yang. “That is what makes our study and the potential benefits of proton therapy so important. We are in Phase 1 of the study, and our initial results are looking promising. Thus far our patients are showing significant tumor reduction without adverse side effects.”

Approximately 60 percent of cancer patients with metastases require radiation. However, the liver can easily be damaged by administering too much radiation. That’s why radiation oncologists are interested in developing advanced treatment options – such as proton therapy – for cancers that have spread to the liver.

Lungs: Non Small Cell Lung Cancer (NSCLC)

Proton therapy reduces side effects such as esophagitis and pneumonitis. I had a good friend die of this disease while I was being treated for my cancer. If only I could have gotten this information to him in time. In one study, women treated with X-rays had a risk of pneumonitis of 14 percent compared to less than one percent risk with proton therapy.

The *International Journal of Radiation Oncolog*y published a study of the National Cancer Database comparing X-rays and protons for Non-Small Cell Lung Cancer (NSCLC) in which proton therapy had higher survival rates. Now, the use of intensity-modulated proton therapy (IMPT) allows even more precision for moving targets such as lung cancer. Surviving cancer is what it’s all about. A higher survival rate is a significant difference.

Yet, despite favorable studies such as this, which number in the hundreds, there are those who drag their feet and claim we need yet more studies to prove whether protons are superior to X-rays. Rather, X-ray radiologists are now scrambling to show that X-rays are as good as protons (but not convincingly so).

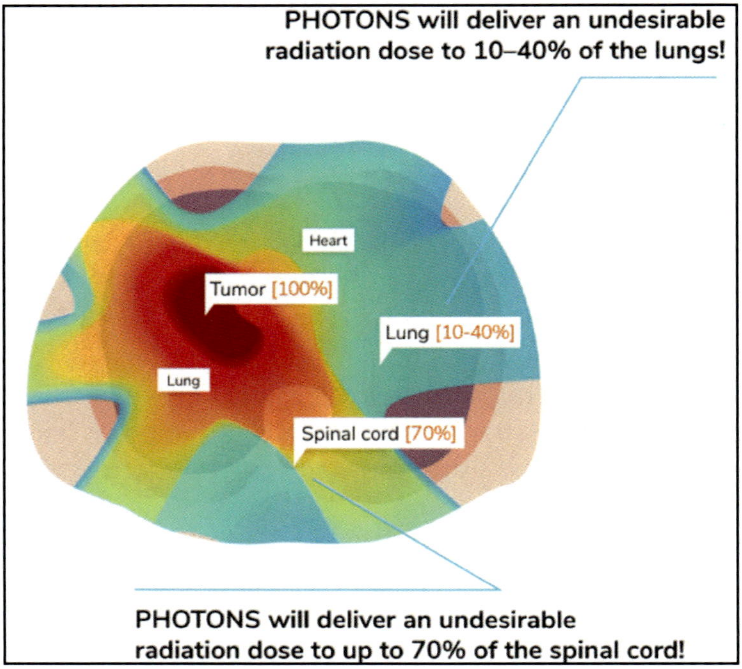

More comparisons.

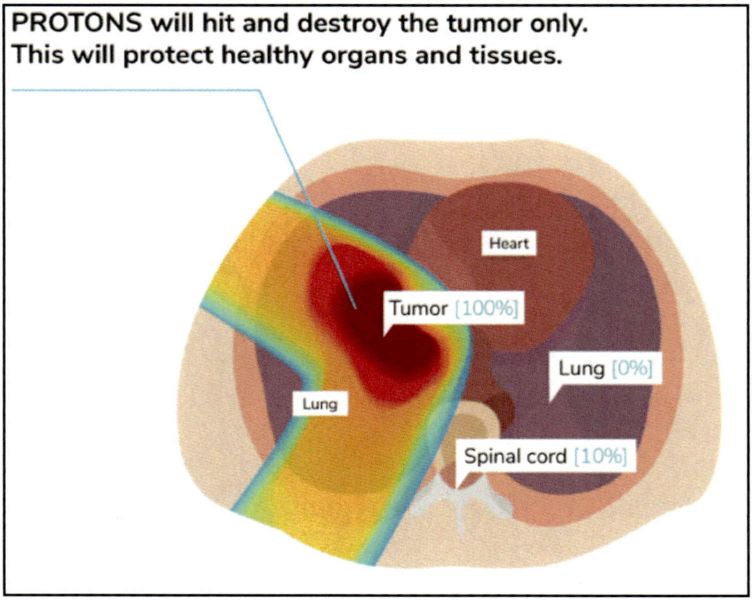

Optical Tumors (ocular melanoma)

The world's first hospital-based proton therapy center was the Clatterbridge Centre for Oncology in the United Kingdom. Opened in 1989, it had a low-energy cyclotron used for ocular tumors. A proton center in Davis, California, also for ocular cancer, opened in 1994.

Because of their accessibility, shallow depth and soft tissue, eyes require very little energy behind the protons. Therefore, the first proton therapy centers to open to the public used equipment that produced only low energy protons, suitable solely for optical purposes. Many proton therapy centers with high-powered cyclotrons cannot reach such a low level. An abstract on PubMed said this about protons and ocular tumors.

Proton beam radiotherapy of uveal melanoma and other malignant and benign ocular tumors has shown tremendous development and success over the past four decades. Proton beam is associated with the lowest overall risk of local tumor recurrence in uveal melanoma, compared with other eye-conserving forms of primary treatment. Proton beam is also utilized for other malignant and benign tumors as primary, salvage, or adjuvant treatment with combined modality therapy. The physical characteristics of proton therapy allow for uniform dose distribution, minimal scatter, and sharp dose fall off making it an ideal therapy for ocular tumors in which critical structures lie in close proximity to the tumor. High radiation doses can be delivered to tumors with relative sparing of adjacent tissues from collateral damage. Proton beam therapy for ocular tumors has resulted in overall excellent chances for tumor control, ocular conservation, and visual preservation.

(For full article, see: "Proton therapy for the management of uveal melanoma and other ocular tumors" at https://www.ncbi.nlm.nih.gov/pubmed/27558251)

Think of how delicate it is to work on the eyes. Here is a description from the Loma Linda proton therapy center:

Uveal melanomas, which are also called choroidal melanomas, are malignant tumors of the eye. Historically, these

tumors have been treated by the complete removal of the eye. However, precise forms of radiation treatment such as proton beam therapy have been used to minimize the need for removal. Protons have been used to treat uveal melanomas since the mid-1970s. Reports reveal control rates greater than 95 percent, with long-term survival consistent with survival rates for patients who have had their diseased eyes removed. Most proton patients have retained useful vision in their treated eyes.
(For more information see: https://protons.com/proton-treatments/other-conditions)

Protons make the difference between night and day, blindness or sight.

Oropharynx cancer

On the internet, I found a study by a whole slew of doctors entitled: "Intensity modulated proton beam therapy (IMPT) versus Intensity modulated photon therapy (IMRT = X-rays) for oropharynx cancer patients – a case matched analysis." Here is their conclusion.

Our results suggest that IMPT (protons) *is associated with reduced rates of feeding tube dependency and severe weight loss without jeopardizing outcome.*
(For the full article, see: https://www.ncbi.nlm.nih.gov/pmc/articles/PMC5474304/)

Proton therapy has some critics who think it's no better than X-rays and is overpriced. Have they looked at any of these articles on PubMed? When you add the cost of recurrence, salvage procedures, and impaired lifestyle with X-rays, the cost of proton therapy evens out over the long term.

Pancreatic Cancer (Adenocarcinoma of the pancreas)

This cancer is so deadly and so hard to treat that just the name causes me to get chills. Many people are dead within months of diagnosis. Mass General Hospital reports these dismal statistics:

There were a total of 145 patients. Thirty-one patients were treated with radical surgery, with a 16% operative mortality, a 5-year crude survival rate of 15%, and a local recurrence rate of 50%. Sixty-two patients were treated with a palliative procedure with a 5-year crude survival of 5%. Fifty-two patients were treated with biopsy alone, with no 5-year survivors.
(See (For full article, see: https://onlinelibrary.wiley.com/doi/abs/10.1002/1097-0142%28197603%2937%3A3%3C1519%3A%3)

What horrible numbers! The standard treatment is surgery followed by radiation. With proton therapy, the kidneys, stomach, and spinal cord can avoid damage, making it possible to give higher doses to help increase the rate of success. I found one PubMed study using proton therapy for recurrences of pancreatic cancer. They concluded that proton therapy was:

. . . well tolerated, resulted in prolonged clinical outcomes compared to historical controls, and should be considered as a treatment option with concurrent chemotherapy in selected patients with locally-recurrent pancreatic cancer.
(See (For full article see: https://www.ncbi.nlm.nih.gov/pubmed/?term=well+tolerated%2C+resulted+in+prolonged+clinical+outcomes+compared+to+historical+controls%2C+and+should+be+considered+as+a+treatment+option+with+concurrent+chemotherapy+in+selected+patients+with+locally-recurrent%C2%A0pancreatic+cancer.)

Amid the medical language, it says that proton therapy patients lived longer than by previous methods. Shall I repeat that? Lived *longer* than by previous methods. Another study said that there was less recurrence with proton therapy and better quality of life, but the survival rate was about the same. It's a bad situation, no matter what, but better quality of life is still something.

Pediatric Cancers

Does anything tug at the heart strings more than seeing children with cancer? How often they are brave and cheerful in the face of devastating side effects. Because of young developing brains and bodies, the long-term effects of X-rays and chemotherapy can greatly decrease their quality of life. Protons for pediatric cancers are widely recognized as the preferred treatment. The cancers treated include brain, pediatric sarcoma, retinoblastoma, neuroblastoma, lymphomas, and any number of rare cancers. On PubMed I found this conclusion:

The present study clearly demonstrates the advantage of conformal radiation methods for the treatment of posterior fossa and spinal column in children with medulloblastoma, when compared to conventional X-rays. Of the two conformal treatment methods evaluated, protons were found to be superior to IMRT.
(See https://www.ncbi.nlm.nih.gov/pubmed/?term=The+present+study+clearly+demonstrates+the+advantage+of+conformal+radiation+methods+for+the+treatment+of+posterior+fossa+and+spinal+column+in+children+with+medulloblastoma.)

St. Jude Children's Research Hospital in Memphis, Tennessee now has proton therapy. So does the Angie Fowler Adolescent & Young Adult Cancer Institute at University Hospital in Cleveland, Ohio and Children's Hospital of Philadelphia (CHOP). I saw children being treated in Knoxville at Provision CARES Proton Therapy Center. The atmosphere is far more family-like and comforting than a big institutional setting.

In 2014 worldwide news accounts followed the dramatic story of five-year-old Ashya King and his family's extreme efforts to have his brain tumor treated with proton therapy. Ashya's story is told in the book *Saving Ashya*, by his mother, Naghmeh King. I have a lengthy book review at the end of this book. It is quite amazing what they went through to get proton therapy and the extent to which the medical community was unhelpful.

Meanwhile, back in the United States, I found the following study from the University of Pennsylvania School of Medicine:

Pediatric patients with head and neck cancer can be treated with proton beam therapy (PBT) instead of traditional photon radiation (X-rays), and it will result in similar outcomes with less impact on quality of life. Researchers from the Perelman School of Medicine at the University of Pennsylvania as well as Children's Hospital of Philadelphia (CHOP) analyzed cases of pediatric head and neck cancer treated with PBT between 2010 and 2016 and found similar rates of tumor control and lower rates of toxicity than what is historically expected from photon radiation. They published their findings in the journal Pediatric Blood and Cancer.

Cancers of the head and neck account for about 12 percent of all pediatric cancers, and they are generally different tumor types than those that affect adults. For solid tumors like neuroblastoma, thyroid cancer, and soft tissue sarcomas, treatment usually involves a combination of therapies including chemotherapy, radiation, and surgery. Post-operative radiation can be critical, since surgeons may not be able to completely remove all cancer given the complexity of the head and neck region.

The area's sensitivity also means the effects of treatment can lower patient quality of life due to symptoms including loss of appetite, difficulty swallowing, or mucositis – in which ulcers form in the digestive tract, usually in reaction to chemotherapy or radiation.

"These concerns are especially important to address in pediatric patients, since they're still developing and may need to deal with any adverse effects for the rest of their lives. This study shows that protons may be an important tool in improving quality of life both during treatment and for years after for these young patients," said the study's senior author Christine Hill-Kayser, MD, chief of the Pediatric Radiation Oncology Service at Penn and an attending physician at CHOP. CHOP cancer patients who need radiation therapy are treated at Penn, including proton therapy through the Roberts Proton Therapy Center.

Jennifer Vogel, MD, a resident in Radiation Oncology at Penn, is the study's lead author. Researchers looked at 69 pediatric head and neck cancer patients treated with PBT (proton beam therapy) *at Penn and CHOP between 2010 and 2016. Thirty-five (50 percent) of those patients had rhabdomyosarcoma, a cancer of the cells that make up skeletal muscles. Ten (7 percent) were treated for Ewing sarcoma, a cancer most commonly found in the bone or soft tissue. The other 24 were treated for a variety of other cancers affecting the head and neck regions.*

One year after treatment, 93 percent of patients were still alive, and 92 percent did not experience recurrence at their primary disease site.

Toxicities, or side effects, are measured on a scale from 1 to 5 with 5 being the most severe. In this study, no patients were above grade 3, and the most severe toxicities at that level were mucositis (4 percent), loss of appetite (22 percent), and difficulty swallowing (7 percent).

"Different disease sites required different dosage levels, and we specifically found the severity of mucositis was associated with higher doses of radiation," Vogel said.

Those numbers are still well below what is typically associated with photon radiation. In rhabdomyosarcoma, for example, 46 percent of patients historically report grade 3 or 4 mucositis.

"These data show proton therapy is not only effective, it is also more tolerable for patients," Hill-Kayser said. "This study shows this treatment is safe and offers practice guidelines for delivering head and neck proton therapy in the pediatric population."

Researchers say they plan to follow up with these patients to evaluate long-term disease control and late-developing toxicity.

October 23, 2017

(From the University of Pennsylvania School of Medicine. See: https://www.sciencedaily.com/releases/2017/10/171023123051.htm).

Pelvic Chondrosarcoma (bone cancer)

I wouldn't have known to include this type of cancer except I got an email in response to one of my blog articles from business consultant and keynote speaker David Bowles, Ph.D. (see www.davidbowlesphd.com). Here's what he said about being treated at the proton therapy center in San Diego:

I had a large hip bone tumor for which I had been offered, by EVERY doctor I talked to except one, a 15 hour surgery which might have left me in a wheelchair for life, with major side effects (deep infection, lymphedema, etc.) to boot. I am now cancer free and totally mobile, thanks to this incredible treatment (proton therapy) and the people who delivered it (beyond the breathtaking technology, treatment planning is an art).

In my case, pelvic chondrosarcoma, and in the cases of the many little kids I saw with brain tumors, with other adults having chordomas and other sarcomas, proton therapy is life-changing and even life-saving. My doctor at the Proton Center, a brilliant guy named Ryan Grover, believes that my recovery from a cancer which had always been treated surgically might just have shown the next generation of pelvic chondrosarcoma patients a completely new path for their treatment. It is early days, but we will see!

He went on to say that Chondrosarcoma isn't affected at all by chemotherapy or regular radiation. Up until now, surgery has been the only option, even though it might cripple the patients for life and leave them with years' worth of negative side effects. Now that may no longer be necessary. David continued.

Surgery has been the standard of care for many years for my cancer. In the old days, they would amputate the limb up to the buttock! So the "newer" version, a hemipelvectomy, is considered "limb sparing." Ha!!! Their view of "success" is that the patient is alive and cancer free after five years. Concerns about quality of life after surgery are downplayed, as several former hemipelvectomy patients on the Facebook Chondrosarcoma page have pointed out.

It's terrible. So I said "no, my view of success is I am mobile and healthy right away and stay that way for as long as possible, and if that's only two years, OK, I prefer that to a decade in a debilitated state, with greatly reduced mobility."

On television pharmaceutical advertisements, in small print at the bottom of the screen, often a line states "individual results may vary." David's tale may be a unique result pioneering the use of proton therapy that hopefully will become standard. I'm just pointing out that's what David did, and, so far, he has survived in great shape. His email spurred me to research on PubMed, where I found the following:

Chondrosarcoma (CS) is a primary malignant bone tumor with cartilaginous differentiation. Poor rates of survival and high rates of local recurrence after surgical treatment have been reported in previous studies. ***The only available treatment*** *is carcinological surgical resection since the usual adjuvant treatments are ineffective. The pelvic location creates*

specific technical difficulties both for exeresis and reconstruction. Our objective was to evaluate the carcinological and functional outcomes of inter-ilioabdominal amputation and conservative surgery.
(For similar articles, see: https://search.nih.gov/search?utf8=%E2%9C%93&affiliate=nih&query=Chondrosarcoma+%28CS%29+is+a+primary+malignant+bone+tumor+with+cartilaginous+differentiation.+Poor+rates+of+survival+and+high+rates+of+local+recurrence+after+surgical+treatment+have+been+reported+in+previous+studies.&commit=Search)

I added the bold emphasis for "the only available treatment" part. That's not true! The results were abysmal for the 59 people in the study. While a small group, the results make my point. If diagnosed with this rare cancer, the prognosis is grim. Here were the results from this group.

Eighteen patients (31%) had a local recurrence, and 12 (20%) had metastases. At last follow-up, 30 patients (51%) were still alive without any sign of recurrence. Twenty-three patients (39%) died from the disease.

The average age of the patients was 48 years. Commonly, the 600 or so people who get this rare bone cancer every year range in age from 20 to 60 years old — not a bunch of old guys as with prostate cancer. People in midlife experienced a 31% failure rate plus another 20% experienced a spread of the cancer while another 39% died from the cancer. In the article, they decry the difficulty of getting a sufficient margin around the cancer (thus the high rate of recurrence). No mention of proton therapy or that surgery is NOT the only available treatment. Protons come riding in like a knight on a white horse, offering hope where there was very little. Alas, the medical community doesn't seem to welcome it, giving patients advice that leads to devastating results, when protons would do such a superior job. I'm not instructing you to ignore your doctor, only to educate him or her and to seek your best option. David had to go to five doctors before finding the solution of proton therapy.

Prostate Cancer

Because prostate cancer is considered easy to treat, some pundits feel proton therapy represents overkill and extra expense. X-rays, they say, are just as good. For that reason, many insurance policies will not cover proton therapy for prostates. (More about insurance issues later.)

Medicare has considered protons for prostate as "Medically Necessary" since 1997. For advanced non-metastatic prostate cancer, protons are an important modality. In January of 2019, United Healthcare begrudgingly agreed to cover proton therapy for prostate cancer. Finally!

A five-year study by the University of Florida found these results:

Researchers report that 99 percent, 94 percent and 74 percent of men with low-, intermediate-, and high-risk prostate cancer, respectively, have no signs of cancer recurrence after five years of follow up. Less than one percent in the cohort experienced serious gastrointestinal side effects and approximately three percent experienced serious urologic side effects.
(For this and similar articles see: https://www.floridaproton.org/about-us/research-portfolio)

Having had intermediate prostate cancer, according to this study, my chances of success are 94%. But this study was done without using pencil beam scanning, which I had, and which is even more accurate. Hence, I feel very good about my prospects. And look at the side effects, ranging from one percent to three percent. If you arrive for treatment already in a weakened state such as having diabetes or being obese, side effects are more likely to occur.

Prostate cancer is the bread and butter of most proton therapy centers. At that 2017 PTCOG-NA conference in Chicago, the following studies were also presented.

Two presentations addressed the treatment of prostate cancer with proton therapy. In a follow up to previous studies utilizing SERR (Surveillance & End Results Registry) and Medicare claims data to compare outcomes between proton therapy and IMRT, physicians from Northwestern Medicine Chicago Proton Center and the University of Florida Health Proton Therapy Institute analyzed a more contemporary and larger population of patients treated with proton therapy and IMRT. The study included patients treated by multiple proton therapy providers from across the country. Compared with the IMRT cohort, the proton patients had a significantly higher 5-year survival rate (94% vs 87%), fewer bladder complications and fewer secondary cancers.

In a direct comparison of clinical outcomes between cohorts of prostate cancer patients treated with IMRT and proton therapy, investigators from the University of Florida Health Proton Therapy Institute and the Mayo Clinic in Arizona found similar complication rates between IMRT and proton therapy, but significantly higher disease control rates with proton therapy for low and intermediate risk prostate cancer patients. Disease control rates for high risk prostate cancer patients were similar between the proton and IMRT cohorts, but hormone therapy was not used as often or for as long a duration in patients who received proton therapy.

Commenting on the studies, Dr. William Hartsell, Medical Director for the Northwestern Medicine Chicago Proton Therapy Center, stated "These studies show the potential for proton therapy to improve outcomes for patients, especially in reducing the side effects from treatment, which may also allow for more effective treatment and better disease control."
(See website: ptcog.ch)

As you know, my personal journey was prostate cancer. Since it can be reached rather easily by X-rays, most insurance companies don't feel proton therapy is necessary. They don't consider side effects as being relevant, but I do.

I wrote a book about my prostate cancer journey entitled *Prostate* Cancer Treatment: Proton Therapy. My medical physicist told me that proton therapy for prostate cancer really shines when it comes to treating the lymph nodes. The following illustration shows my actual lymph nodes (and other organs) as outlined in the RaySeach software. Proton therapy only became viable when scanning and software technologies provided the visibility and planning assistance critical to this kind of complexity.

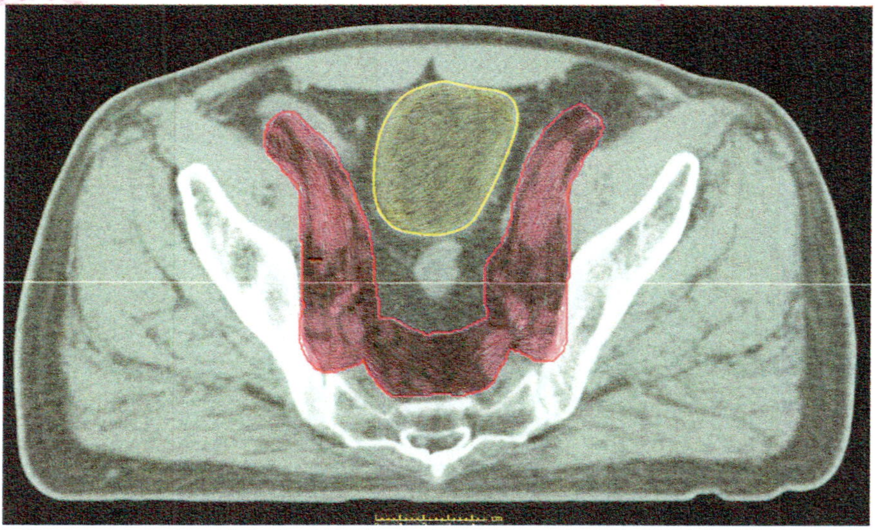

Here is a picture of my lymph nodes (maroon color) that form a "U" shape around the bladder (yellow) and rectum. The large white areas are bone.

Protons can treat each lymph area separately, left and right, which is exactly how I was treated. The protons were beamed on one side, and then I was turned around to treat the other side. X-rays would go all the way across, affecting the bladder and rectum, which are located in the middle.

My protons were delivered through the femur heads whereas X-rays would be directed from numerous directions, thereby irradiating healthy tissue.

As we have said before, both X-rays and protons kill the cancer. The difference lies in damage to healthy tissue and quality of life issues.

When I put out a request for illustrations for this book, I waited for several months to no avail. Finally, I contacted the proton therapy center in Prague, which came to my rescue in a matter of days. I am very appreciative of their kindness. On the next page are some more of their materials pertaining to prostate cancer.

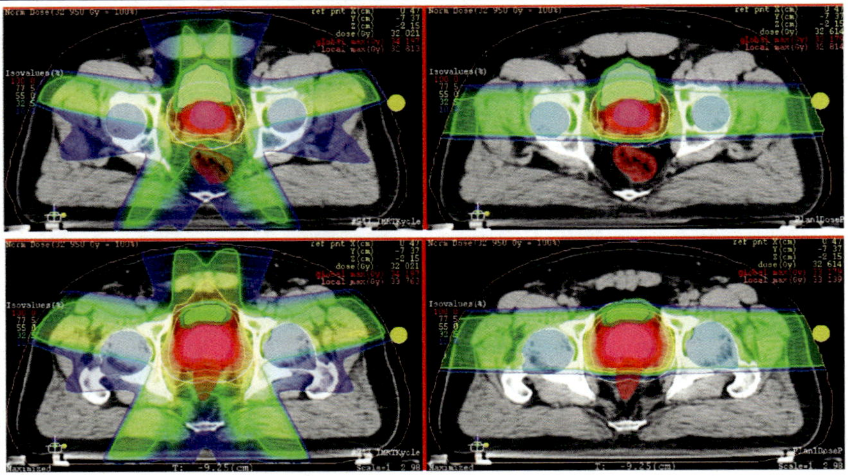

Prostate IMRT (left) IMPT @ 5% isodose

X-rays, shown on the left, would affect far more healthy tissue than protons, shown on the right.

Below is a chart pertaining to side effects of treatment. The numbers may vary from one study to another, but they are always in the same order. Surgery is the worst (on the left), X-rays are in the middle, and protons have the least effect (on the right). The three groups below illustrate impotence, incontinence, and relapse (recurrence).

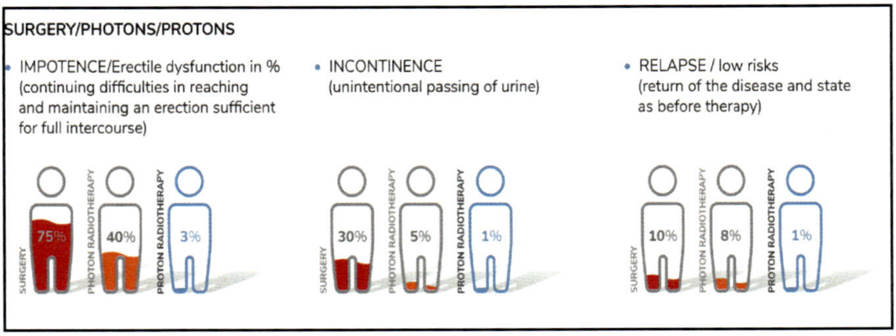

KUBES, Jiri, Tereza HRCIAROVA and Tomas DOLEZAL. Toxicity after prostate tumour irradiation with proton beams: Regimen 36.25 Gray (5 x 7.25). Proton Therapy Center in Prague, 2017.

Recurrent Tumors

When a cancer treatment fails and the cancer must again be addressed, that's called a salvage procedure. With proton therapy, salvage procedures can deal with the recurrence of most cancers, despite how it was first treated. Often, after surgery, scar tissue makes additional surgery more difficult. As we noted with the center in Prague, they have a whole specialty of dealing with failed cancer treatments.

A study in the United Kingdom found that out of every 1,000 new cancer patients, 523 (52%) are given radiation therapy as part of their treatment. Unfortunately, out of these, 120 patients (23%) will require re-treatment. This startling number refers to all cancers. Protons come into play in two ways. First, they have less recurrent cancer and secondly, they can be used to treat most types of recurrent cancer.

Skin Cancer

As I researched various kinds of cancer treated by proton therapy, I wondered if it could be used for skin cancer. I came across an article in the newsletter from the proton center in Seattle about a man with exactly such a case. Here is what it said.

Merkel cell carcinoma is typically a fast-growing, painless nodule on the skin and can appear as flesh-colored or in shades of red, blue or purple bumps on the face, head or neck. This type of skin cancer is about 40 times rarer than melanoma. It is aggressive, tending to grow quickly, and can rapidly spread to other parts of the body even with treatment, which is why early diagnosis is extremely important.

His doctors decided that in addition to surgery, radiation or chemotherapy would be needed. One of his doctors recommended that radiation would be best, and that proton therapy would be the best kind of radiation, because of its ability to precisely focus the radiation to the exact location of the cancer cells.

(See full article in newsletter here: https://www.sccaprotontherapy.com/survivor-stories/stories/jim-200218.)

Besides its capacity as a stand alone treatment, proton therapy can also be used in conjunction with chemotherapy or, in this case, surgery, to track down every last bit of cancer.

Spinal Cord Tumors (Intradural tumor)

A spinal cord tumor, also called an intradural tumor, is a spinal tumor that begins within the spinal cord or the covering of the spinal cord (dura). A tumor that affects the bones of the spine (vertebrae) is called a vertebral tumor.

Spinal cord tumors are classified differently depending on where they occur relative to the protective membranes of the spinal cord. These are the main types of intradural tumors: Intramedullary tumors begin in the cells within the spinal cord itself, such as gliomas, astrocytomas, or ependymomas. Extramedullary tumors grow in either the membrane surrounding the spinal cord or the nerve roots that reach out from the spinal cord. Although they don't begin within the spinal cord itself, these types of tumors may affect spinal cord function by causing spinal cord compression and other problems. Examples of extramedullary tumors that can affect the spinal cord include meningiomas, neurofibromas, schwannomas, and nerve sheath tumors.

Intensity modulated proton therapy (IMPT) lets radiation oncologists adjust the precision, depth, and intensity of a proton beam to the peaks and valleys of complex spider-like tumors while avoiding healthy tissue. Tumors like these are typically found in the head, neck or spine.

* * *

The above list of cancer types treatable with proton therapy is not exhaustive. For all cancers, the principles are the same: more accurate, less damage to healthy tissues, fewer side effects, better quality of life. I hope this is a convincing demonstration for the reader to look into the possibilities of proton therapy.

5

HOW PROTONS KILL CANCER

Protons damage both cancerous cells and healthy cells in the same way. They damage the DNA by ionizing it, taking away electrons to balance the positively charged protons. Healthy cells can recover whereas cancer cells do not due to their instability. Spreading out the fractions allows healing to take place in surrounding tissue.

Suppose both cancerous and healthy cells start at level ten (a measurement I have made up for illustrative purposes). Proton treatment reduces them to six. The healthy cells bounce back to ten but the cancer cells only to nine. After the next treatment, the healthy cells recover to ten again, but the cancer cells only to eight. After the next treatment, the healthy cells go back to ten but the cancer cells only to seven. The cancer reaches a threshold level below which it can no longer recover or reproduce. The healthy tissue returns to normal.

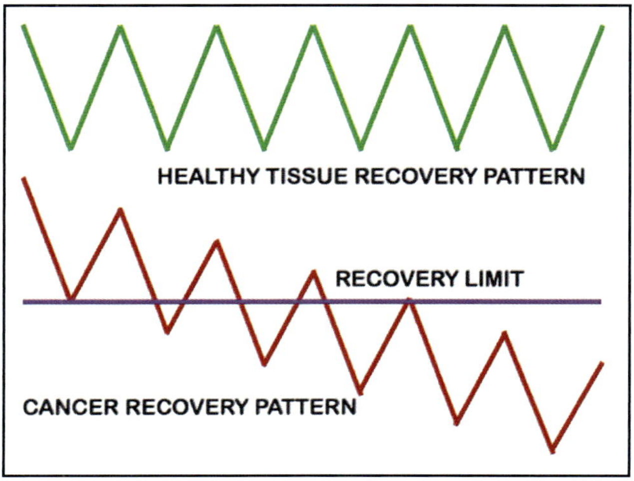

I made the above diagram to summarize the recovery process of both types of cells. What it doesn't show is time. The destruction of the cancer cells continues over time, long after the proton treatment ends. I was told that for two years after having prostate cancer the PSA will be an unreliable indicator as the process takes its course. That being said, my first post-treatment test went from 16.0 down to 1.4. Now, more than three years later, it is 0.3.

I have read that the most effective way to disable cancer cells and thus prevent their reproduction is to cause a double-strand break in the DNA. Remember that protons have mass, where as x-rays do not. To the DNA, protons are like wrecking balls. As a result, a number of studies have shown that protons cause far more double-strand breaks than do photons.

Just because protons are superior in treating these types of cancers doesn't mean they will be used for that purpose. There are barriers. One is the lack of knowledge about protons. Another is the refusal of insurance companies to cover it. A third is conflicting advice given by the medical community.

Consider John McCain, who was diagnosed and treated for glioblastoma. Not surprisingly, he was treated at the Mayo Clinic in Phoenix. They have proton therapy capability, but I read nothing indicating they used it. Why not, I wonder?

In my hometown of San Antonio, I gave a talk about proton therapy attended by a man who had developed brain cancer. He went to MD Anderson in Houston, where he received treatment with X-rays that damaged his brain and left him with serious cognitive impairment. They have a proton therapy center at MD Anderson, which could have avoided that result. He asked me after the talk why they hadn't treated his brain cancer with protons. My guess is that his family doctor didn't know about proton therapy and referred him to a radiologist who specialized in X-rays. It's very easy to get cynical and angry when the medical community does not seem to give us the best treatment, but rather, the most profitable one for them. Healthcare for profit doesn't serve us well.

6
CRITICISM

When searching for information about proton therapy, you are likely to run across some sources that are critical. Amitabh Chandra, director of health policy research at the Harvard Kennedy School of Government is one such critic. Because of his elevated position, he is quoted widely. Ironically, it was at Harvard that proton therapy was developed for more than fifty years. Yet Chandra has said:

I view proton-beam therapy as ground zero to look at whether we are going to bend the cost curve. It's very hard to spot waste in healthcare. Proton therapy is an example of waste you can spot right away. . . . Nothing so big and so useless has ever been discovered in medicine.

He has compared proton-therapy to the Death Star from Star Wars. Proton therapy useless? And he's the director of health policy? Lordy Lordy. I find his comments ignorant.

Another critic states, "The higher price would be worth it if proton beam therapy cured more people or significantly reduced side effects. But there is no evidence showing this is true." A different article declares, "Despite lack of evidence, more proton beam centers on the way." Still another calls it "crazy medicine and unsustainable public policy."

The critics are wrong. There is plenty of evidence as to the benefits of proton therapy. The mainstream medical community fuels much of this criticism. Critics are dedicated to the status quo. Their most common criticism is that proton therapy is no better, and it costs more, so it's a bad deal. In these pages, I have quoted just a few of the hundreds of favorable studies. I could fill a whole book with them. Everyone acknowledges that proton therapy is expensive, but look at the complexity of both the equipment and the process. And prices are coming down.

A couple of years ago there were several articles carried in the New York Times that were deliberately antagonistic to proton therapy. I see them quoted often. It's not just that they pointed out some of the bumps in the road, of which there have been plenty, but rather, the choice of vocabulary that created an artificial and needless negativity. I wrote two long rebuttals that are available on my blog. (See www.proton-beam-therapy.com.) This article describes greedy developers jacking up the price, over estimating anticipated volume, bankruptcies, and underperformance.

To a small degree, all these have indeed happened, but they are overblown and do not accurately represent the proton therapy industry. These issues are common for any new technology. Further, these issues do not address the excellence of the treatment itself. The most egregious criticism is that proton therapy is over rated and no better than other modalities. My fear is that undue negativity will drive people away from protons when they might be just the right treatment for them. Misinformation can lead to bad decisions, which in turn lead to pain and suffering. We're not talking about choosing the right cellphone here. Cancer threatens our very existence..

Criticism falls into several categories:

1. Those who pontificate while knowing little about the subject
2. Purveyors of other treatments being defensive and protective
3. Defenders of the status quo
4. Would-be muckraking journalists who miss the mark
5. Legitimate, well-informed neutral parties with evidence against proton therapy.

I just made up the fifth category. I don't know of any such criticism. Rather, criticism usually sounds like this:

Proton radiotherapy "sells hope," but there is no "clear measurable benefit that we can actually translate and explain to a patient," said Frank H. Saran, MD, from the Royal Marsden NHS Foundation Trust in the United Kingdom.
(Proton Therapy 'Sells Hope': No Clear Benefit for Patients - Medscape - Jun 20, 2013.)

Dr. Saran had no opportunity to translate and explain proton therapy at all, actually, as in 2013, when this was written, there were no proton centers in the United Kingdom. So the critic had no first-hand knowledge or experience.

X-rays used to be the standard for radiation treatment. When protons first came on the scene, the question was whether they would be as effective as X-rays. Now, X-ray providers are scrambling to show that X-rays are as good as proton therapy.

The American Society of Radiation Oncology (ASTRO) has 10,000 members, most of whom use X-rays. Back in 2009, ASTRO published an article stating that proton therapy isn't any better than less expensive alternatives, such as X-rays. Using that reference as their rationale, Aetna, United Healthcare, and Cigna mostly stopped covering proton therapy. Not being covered by insurance has been a big road block for proton therapy, which in turn, has helped X-ray radiologists keep their clients. Their criticism was clearly self-serving.

Fast forward to May of 2016 when the Red Journal, the 500-page publication of ASTRO, released a special edition about proton therapy. Yes, there was still an article by a holdout radiologist who said he got equal or better results using X-rays, but the rest of the articles were either very technical or overtly positive regarding the potential of protons. Yet, insurance companies still quote the original article and ignore more recent data.

One website I found touted the combination of 4D IG-IMRT utilizing DART and PD-103 brachytherapy, SonArray, Cone Beam Tomography, Exact Couch™, Portal Vision, On-Board Imaging, and Respiratory Gating, concluding "None of this is even remotely possible with protons." I would respond that it is not remotely *necessary* with protons.

In the 2020 edition of this book, I have shortened this chapter. I was trying to refute every kind of criticism. Instead let me go into some detail about two typical examples.

From the website of Cyberknife and Radiation Oncology Center in Phoenix, Arizona I found this:

The Annals of Internal Medicine conducted a comprehensive literature review of proton radiation therapy where they reviewed 243 articles on 185 studies that included 17 clinical trials. The findings from the literature review was that no comparative study reported statistically significant differences in survival-rates or adverse effects in proton therapy versus IMRT. From analyzing these sources, we find that there is no proven benefit or statistical difference in tumor control, adverse effects, or dosimetry when using proton beam radiation therapy versus IMRT.

(See website: http://phoenixcyberknifecenter.com/proton-therapy/.)

Besides noting the grammatical errors, I was concerned when I read this, as it refers to one of the most prestigious medical journals in the world. So, I looked up the study. First, it said that there are only seven proton therapy centers, which dates it considerably (at least ten years old). The conclusion stated above comes from this sentence: "No comparative study reported statistically significant or important differences in overall or cancer-specific survival or in total serious adverse events." That seems to say protons were not statistically better. But let's read the next several sentences:

"Limitation: Few studies directly compared treatments with or without particle irradiation." Oh, so there weren't 243 studies that directly compared protons to X-rays. There were only a few. Then this: "Conclusion: Evidence on the comparative effectiveness and safety of charged-particle radiation therapy (proton therapy) in cancer is needed to assess the benefits, risks, and costs of treatment alternatives."

The study actually says that more evidence is needed to make a proper assessment. Misquoting conclusions is one way to produce authentic-sounding criticism. Another way is to build bias into the study itself.

The next example is so troublesome that I have written an entire blog about it entitled "Proton Critics Cling to Flawed Study." A study from MD Anderson and Massachusetts General Hospital was described in MedPage Today under the following headline: "No Reduced Toxicity for Proton Tx vs IMRT in NSCLC." Proton Tx stands for proton treatment. IMRT is Intensity-Moderated

Radiation Therapy, a type of X-ray treatment. NSCLC stands for Non-Small Cell Lung Cancer. The purpose of study was not to determine the effectiveness in killing the cancer. Rather, it measured damage to tissues. The study concedes that proton therapy exposes less heart tissue to radiation than x-rays, but that wasn't their focus.

Yet, what if it were? Suppose they were measuring heart exposure. Then, the headline would have been "Proton Therapy Exposes Heart to Less Damage than IMRT." I think that would be extremely relevant to the patient. Instead, they were measuring radiation pneumonitis, inflammation of the lungs caused by radiation. After one year, the combined rates of toxicity were 17.4% for IMRT and 21.1% for proton therapy. X-rays win, or so it would seem. Reading only this conclusion critics quote this study profusely to show proton therapy is no better than X-rays when it comes to side effects. Except for one problem. **The study actually showed just the opposite**.

First, the proton technology used was the older PSPT (passively scattered proton therapy) technique, and not the more up-to-date pencil beam scanning. So they are making a judgement about all proton therapy based on its lesser version. So this study compares the best form of X-rays with a lesser form of proton therapy. That's because it took place in 2012, though the article about the results was in 2018. Old.

The design of the study called for protons and X-rays to do the same thing. Hence, protons were treating some lymph nodes from the opposite side of the chest which, like the X-rays, did indeed cause pneumonitis. That's typical for X-rays, but protons don't need to do that. Proton therapy can and should treat the patients from the near side without damage. After the experimenters had learned more about using protons, they changed and radiated the lymph nodes from the near side of the patient. Question: Why is this considered a major finding when those running the trial didn't know what they were doing? It looks like on-the-job training, learning as they go.

For the second half of the study, after treating the lymph nodes from the closest side, the incidence of pneumonitis caused by proton therapy was reduced to zero. Zero! For IMRT, the rate stayed the same because the experimenters were already using X-rays expertly. During the second half of the trial, then, the actual side effects were zero for proton therapy and 6.5% for IMRT. Had they used protons correctly in the first half, the results would have been as overwhelming for the whole study as they were for the second half.

In stead, the conclusion gave figures for the whole trial, allowing the early statistics to drag down and dilute the real results achieved later in the study. Thus, it appeared that protons did poorly when just the opposite is true. The inequality gets even worse.

Dr. Jeffrey Bradley from the proton therapy center in St. Louis, Missouri, examined the study and said this:

So by design, they tried to give the same radiation dose to both arms, but you've taken away an advantage of proton beam therapy, because allowing a higher dose with protons is one of the advantages of the technology. Let's say you had an ice hockey team, and you can't use your best skaters--everybody on the team has to be able to skate at the same level. You know you're going to get a similar outcome. Almost all experts in proton radiation therapy feel like they handicapped themselves by that study design.

By using protons as if they were X-rays, their real strength (their best players) was not allowed. The study had a flawed basis from the very beginning. Plus they used an older, version of proton therapy, reporting their findings six years later after the initiation of pencil beam scanning. Dr. Bradley explains more.

"In addition, the targets were larger on the proton arm than they were on the IMRT arm. It was early in the proton experience and they were worried about missing the target so they enlarged their aperture. They ended up treating, circumferentially, about 8-10 mm wider around the tumor with the proton arm. We've learned not to do that."

So lets review. Despite an older technology, questionable trial design, unskilled application, dose restrictions, and an enlarged target, protons still performed far better than X-rays once the technicians learned how to do it.

After the study had been released, others commented on it including Dr. Feng-Ming (Spring) Kong, MD, from the Indiana University School of Medicine, who wrote an editorial about this study entitled "What Happens When Proton Meets Randomization: Is There a Future for Proton Therapy?" Just the title gives me pause. Does the future of proton therapy rest with this one flawed trial? She said this:

Completion of this study is not trivial because the evaluation of the benefit of a new technology rarely has been done during the century-long history of radiation oncology practice. . . Linac-based three-dimensional conformal technology and the current widespread use of IMRT technologies have been developed and implemented routinely in the clinic without randomized trials.

Excuse me? Radiologists are clamoring for randomized trials for proton therapy when the technology they themselves use was itself never subjected to this kind of scrutiny! Then, Dr. Kong makes a very cogent observation.

Some may even argue that conducting a trial to test the significance of such a treatment is unethical, like performing a randomized study to test the value of parachutes, because it will put patients at risk for unneeded radiation complications.

Great analogy. How would you like to be in the group with the inferior parachutes? Or X-rays? Many intended studies comparing X-rays and protons don't take place because they can't find willing participants. No one wants the X-rays.

Then, somewhat ingenuously, Dr, Kong makes this conclusion. *"Whether a better planning technique such as proton intensity modulation (IMPT) or pencil beam scanning (PBS) would have generated different results is hard to predict."* No, it isn't hard to predict; protons would do even better. Dr. Kong comes from a medical center that has X-rays but not proton therapy. She admits ". . . *the study design in terms of end point definition, control of confounding factors, and dealing with the lung dosimetric restriction may have confounded the results."* Exactly! The design of the study and the performance of those who conducted it skewed the results. Intentionally? One wonders. Still, she shows her allegiance to X-rays by stating, *"Personally, as a radiation oncologist, I would not recommend proton therapy for NSCLC outside a clinical trial setting until a clinical benefit is demonstrated in a prospective randomized study."*

In other words, this *wasn't* a prospective randomized trial? Boo, hiss. Did she fail to notice proton therapy did show benefits? How, then, could she write an editorial about it? As we see frequently, although proton therapy came out on top, its critics still demand more studies.

Proton therapy has to endure this type of prejudice, but it won't stop their progress. In other studies, the patients recruited for X-rays were well-suited but the ones for proton therapy were problematic; again creating an unfair comparison. Currently, there are several well-funded double blind studies comparing proton therapy pencil beam scanning with IMRT. Again, they are having problems getting participants. The results to date look favorable for proton therapy.

I have taken all this space to give the reader enough knowledge to evaluate faulty criticism. Much of it comes from a handful of journalists. The journalistic tradition of muckraking originated in investigative reporting in the early twentieth century exposing corruption and injustices. That's a good thing. However, several journalists have decided they need to protect the public from the evils of proton therapy. To make a living, they repeatedly publish articles using the same biased sources and expressing the same mistaken conclusions.

Some criticism is helpful, clarifying ways in which proton therapy can and should be improved. These are mostly found in scientific journals, and can be worthwhile. Meanwhile, don't be dissuaded by negative things you may read. Go right to the source. Look at the websites of some of the proton therapy centers. Be proactive; get the facts.

7

INSURANCE

Cost and coverage, the two big C's, continue to impede the progress of proton therapy. I have written extensively about insurance matters in my other books, and especially on my blog (www.proton-beam-therapy.com). The crux of the matter is that proton therapy is hugely expensive and insurance companies don't want to pay. Criticism, too, is often not about effectiveness but excessive cost, which critics feel keeps protons from being a good value.

A study by MD Anderson of insurance suppliers in Texas found a wide range of definitions of medical necessity and insurance coverage. Each company seemed to follow its own policy. Every proton therapy center has staff members dedicated solely to getting and managing insurance coverage. I went to Provision CARES Proton Therapy Center in Knoxville largely because of their expertise with insurance.

My United Healthcare AARP Secure Horizons Advantage plan made it clear that they would *not* pay for proton therapy for prostate cancer. In January, 2019, they changed that policy after some highly visible large judgements against insurance companies for wrongly refusing to cover proton therapy.

I went to Provision because I could join a study, called a registry, which will track me for life to verify the effectiveness of proton therapy. The study isn't just for prostate cancer it's for all types of cancer treated with protons. Because I joined the registry, Medicare paid 80% of the cost of my treatment. Provision then got United Healthcare to cover the other 20%. In that way, I dodged the insurance bullet. This seemed too good to be true, so I went to the medicare website to see for myself. I found that Provision had it right. Medicare does have a registry that will pay for your treatment. There are many trials and studies out there, but few of them pay for the treatment as Medicare does.

Clinical Research studies
<u>How often is it covered?</u>
Medicare covers clinical research studies which test different types of medical care, like how well a cancer drug works. These studies help doctors and researchers see if a new treatment works and is safe. Medicare Part A (Hospital Insurance) and/or Medicare Part B (Medical Insurance) cover some costs, like office visits and tests and in certain qualifying clinical research studies.
<u>Who's eligible?</u>
All people with Part A and Part B are covered in qualifying studies.
<u>Your Costs in Original Medicare</u>
You may have to pay 20% of the Medicare-approved amount depending on the treatment you get. The Part B deduction may apply.
Medicare will help pay for some of your costs if you join a covered clinical research study.

Read that last sentence again. Music to my ears.

Anyone on Medicare can get proton therapy if they agree to be on this registry and meet the qualifications. Such registries are administered regionally, so it is necessary to check with each proton center to ascertain whether they participate in such a registry. My total cost, for a few non-covered items, copays, and living in Knoxville for two months came to about $12,000.

Medicare covers cancers listed in Group I. For other cancers, in Group II, you must be in a registry or clinical trial to get covered. Here is a quotation directly from Medicare material:

Group 2 indications define conditions that are still under investigation and may be covered when the LCD criteria are met.

LCD stands for Local Coverage Determination. This is determined by the regional MAC (Medicare Administrative Contractor), an independent contractor who administers coverage and payment for Medicare. The MAC for Provision is Cahaba Government Benefit Administrators, LLC, whose geographical area includes Alabama, Georgia, and Tennessee. Registries and trials cover a wide range of cancers, including the following:

1. Unresectable lung cancers and upper abdominal/peri-diaphragmatic cancers.
2. Advanced stage, unresectable pelvic tumors including those with peri-aortic nodes or malignant lesions of the cervix.
3. Unresectable breast tumors in proximity to the heart.
4. Unresectable pancreatic and adrenal tumors.
5. Skin cancer with microscopic perineural/cranial nerve invasion of the skull base.
6. Unresectable malignant lesions of the liver, bilary tract, anal canal and rectum.
7. Prostate cancer, non-metastatic.

Unresectable refers to a malignancy that can't be surgically removed, due either to metastatic foci or location in a surgical danger zone. Protons, however, can reach those areas.

If you would like proton therapy but are not old enough for Medicare coverage, I suggest investigating the possibility of having your treatment paid for by the party doing a trial. Go to this website: www.clinicaltrials.gov. The last time I checked it showed 317,735 studies from fifty states and 209 countries. My search under proton therapy yielded 715 studies.

I have been told directly by several centers that they have been quite successful in getting coverage for proton therapy. In Florida, for example, and in California at the center in Loma Linda. I received an email from the Loma Linda University Medical Center (LLUMC) stating the following:

Offsetting the costs of proton therapy is a primary concern for both patients and LLUMC. This is why the Proton Treatment Center accepts insurance plans from 250 providers including Medicare and Medicaid. While most medical insurers will consider proton treatment on a case-by-case basis, our financial coordinators will provide further assistance in coordinating these sensitive financial matters. Our financial coordinators can assist you in working with your insurance company to obtain authorization.

Loma Linda, being the first proton center, got the best website (protons.com) and toll-free number (1-800-protons). Easy to remember. They assured me that they do well with insurance companies. I suspect insurance companies always say no, perhaps through several levels of appeal, weeding out those claimants who aren't persistent. When they are dealing with an experienced entity such as LLUMC, however, they know it will pursue the best possible coverage. In such instances, insurance companies cooperate a little more. The proton center in San Diego describes three possible scenarios.

- Full coverage: In most cases, proton therapy is covered by Medicare (non-HMO). Patients covered by private insurance or Medicare supplemental insurance often incur few or no net out-of-pocket expenses after deductibles, copays/coinsurance and annual maximum payments are met.
- Case-by-case coverage: Some insurance plans consider proton therapy on a case-by-case basis. In this situation, our team of specialists work directly with your insurance plan to seek authorization for care by providing appropriate documentation to support the medical necessity of treatment.
- No coverage: For those without insurance, and for international patients without insurance coverage in the United States, the center also offers reduced self-pay options and payment plans.
(For new proton center in San Diego, see: http://www.californiaprotons.com/.)

But suppose you don't qualify for a trial or registry and you are not yet Medicare age. If your insurance company won't cover proton therapy, you must go through a series of appeals. Here are the ways Provision helps with insurance.

"We believe it's important for patients to be empowered to fight for the coverage they deserve when facing a cancer diagnosis," says Rhonda Turner, manager of financial services at Provision Center for Proton Therapy. "We know that we won't always win every case, but together we can improve our chances for success."

Provision assists in the insurance process by providing a letter of medical necessity, making peer-to-peer review calls, crafting individualized appeals, and taking them through multiple levels including external reviews, and offering guidance through any patient appeals or grievance procedures. All proton centers will be equipped to offer this level of service.

You can help your own situation by filing a patient grievance letter, organizing a conference call between the proton center and your insurer, or contacting your employer, as some employers can override insurance coverage decisions

At Provision patients also help in the fight for others, writing letters to insurance providers, sharing their stories on social media and contacting elected officials. "Public pressure is the best way to ensure coverage of proton therapy in the future," Turner says. "Nobody can communicate the need for proton therapy better than those who are being denied access to it."
See more at: http://provisionproton.com/blog/page/2/#sthash.reFNLO3g.dpuf

You can also:
- Contact your insurance company and ask for information about how to appeal at a higher level or to another entity.
- Consider seeking help from one of the many nonprofit and for-profit entities that offer advice. Many states have health insurance consumer advocates.
- Talk to others who have had the same diagnosis and sought treatment with proton therapy.
- Search for success stories online about patients who used proton therapy to treat similar conditions.
- Share your story on social media outlets to publicize your efforts and locate others who may be able to help you.

And, you can sue your insurance company. The most successful cases have either been after the fact, where the patient paid out of pocket and then sued for reimbursement, or by a spouse after the patient died. Legal action has been the newest front opened in the battle for proton therapy. There have been several high-profile cases that have led to large judgements against insurance companies.

I have written about taking legal action is some detail in several of my blogs, including providing source material and arguments to be used by attorneys (www.proton-beam-therapy.com/blog.html). If denying proton therapy costs insurance companies more through judgements than to cover the treatment, perhaps they will change.

"It is undisputed among legitimate medical experts that proton radiation therapy is not experimental and causes much less collateral damage than traditional radiation. To deny a patient this treatment, if it is available, is immoral and barbaric." This unequivocal statement from U. S. District Judge Robert Scola in Florida went viral in the legal and proton therapy communities.

It followed on the heels of a 25.5 million dollar judgement against Aetna for denying proton therapy. That case was well-suited for a challenge. Doctors at MD Anderson declared that proton therapy was the only treatment that could save the life of the patient. Aetna's position seemed to be driven by the Clinical Policy Bulletins (CPBs), which state their particular stance for coverage or lack thereof.

The studies they used to determine their policy were woefully dated and insufficient. The decision to deny was made by people who knew nothing about proton therapy, following company policy instead of deciding the case on its merits.

A few months later, seeing the writing on the wall, United Healthcare changed its position and said it would cover proton therapy for prostate cancer. Better late than never.

If you Google "insurance coverage for proton therapy" you will find much advice. The main issue is that insurance companies say proton therapy is new and unproven or not medically necessary. Every proton center has dealt with this resistance at great length. They help supply the documentation, as well as guide you through the various levels of appeal.

Thomas R. Bortfeld and Jay S. Loeffler have written:

And in the United States, major insurance companies are denying proton therapy to up to 30% of eligible patients on the basis that there are too few rigorously designed and completed clinical trials providing evidence of better outcomes. In our experience, however, this is a vicious cycle: such trials are difficult to conduct when patients are denied private health

coverage.
(See: https://www.nature.com/news/three-ways-to-make-proton-therapy-affordable-1.22660)

I frequently receive emails from people asking how they can get proton therapy when their insurance company is resistant. Here's what I tell them.

1. Fight back. Be persistent. You will need the assistance of your doctor and other professionals.

2. Are you old enough to be on Medicare? If so, find a proton center that participates in a Medicare registry, as I did, in which Medicare pays 80% of the cost whether your insurance company covers proton therapy or not.

3. Shop around for cost. The University of Florida in Jacksonville quoted the out-of-pocket cost of proton therapy for prostate cancer as $134,000. Provision charges $93,000, for the very same treatment. Better, actually, as their equipment is more advanced. One strategy to win your insurance company over might be to agree to get treatment at the least expensive proton center.

4. A few centers charge the same for proton therapy as for X-rays. This is true, I believe, for the two Mayo Clinic centers (Phoenix AZ and Rochester MN), the University of Pennsylvania, and the University of Maryland centers. If proton therapy didn't cost more than X-rays, insurance companies might approve treatment.

5. Go abroad. If you are paying for treatment yourself, it is cheaper to go abroad. I almost went to Prague to the very excellent center there. They were going to charge $33,000. With travel and lodging, I estimated the cost to be $40,000.

The main thing is to really get in there and fight for your options. Here are some resources for getting help:

http://allianceforprotontherapy.org/

This is an organization founded to help get insurance coverage for proton therapy. They have both success stories and failures. Maybe they can help you.

http://www.proton-therapy.org/howit.htm

This is the National Association for Proton Therapy. They have an extensive section on insurance coverage.

www.proton-therapy-centers.com

This is one of my websites. It lists proton therapy centers, along with addresses, phone numbers, and websites.

www.provosionproton.com

This is the website for Provision, where I was treated. They did a great job with the insurance.

Even when the cost of proton therapy is lower, insurance companies have balked at coverage, perhaps feeling that their cost avoidance would be exposed. Sometimes, they have even broken the law in refusing to pay for treatment. These laws were passed by states concerned that proton therapy was being held to a higher standard of proof than other modalities. The proton center in Hampton, Virginia sued insurance companies to gain equal treatment. Oklahoma passed such a law, as did Tennessee.

We're not alone in facing issues with insurance coverage for proton therapy. In England, where they have universal healthcare, the National Health Service (NHS) determines treatments and pays for them. Or not. Their reluctance to approve proton therapy has led to several celebrated cases. One was Alex Vincent who as a young child was diagnosed with a brain tumor. Doctors at the NHS gave him an 80% likelihood of dying, and even if he survived, conventional treatment might have left him blind, deaf, and in a wheelchair. Being only four years old, he would have sustained serious damage to his still developing body.

Alex's father tells his story:

"I remember in 2008, googling 'anaplastic ependymoma' and I found this link to a hospital in Massachusetts, offering proton beam therapy. It said on the link it was the way forward for babies, toddlers and small children. So I told the specialist in Britain I wanted to take Alex to America for proton therapy treatment rather than having radiotherapy here. He just said: 'It

isn't tried and tested.' He warned us that if we took Alex to the States, we were putting his life in danger. Then he added: 'And anyway, they are probably only after your money.' But I just stuck to my guns."

After the family scrambled to raise the money, Alex was treated in the United States, first surgery, then proton therapy (received in Jacksonville, Florida). His father reports:

"While we were in Florida, all the things the British doctors had told me proton therapy wasn't good for – all these different tumours – actually, it turned out, could be treated with it. The doctors here in the UK had said it was only good for tumours at the base of the back of the neck. That wasn't the case. The proton treatment is good for lots of different tumours."

Today Alex is in excellent health, no thanks to the NHS. The family founded an inspiring website called Alex's Lemonade Stand Foundation, named after one of the activities for raising money. See: https://www.alexslemonade.org/childhood-cancer/type/brain-tumor.

A more recent case involves Ashya King, also with a brain tumor, also given poor advice by the NHS. University Hospital Southampton had already concluded that proton therapy would have "no significant benefit" over the standard course of treatment of X-rays, a view it said was supported by a national independent expert body. The risk of sending the boy abroad, and presumably the cost of doing so, they said, were not worth it. I tell the story at the end of this book in a book review. The parents went through a harrowing experience.

Recently, several proton therapy centers have opened in the UK; so perhaps the NHS will change its policy. I have stressed that I am not giving medical advice in this book. That should be left to the medical establishment. Unfortunately, they frequently give poor advice, as we have seen in the above illustrations. By knowing more ourselves, we are better qualified to get involved in making the right decision.

8

MAKING THE NUMBERS WORK

Proton therapy has such a promising future that the early developers seemed justified in spending hundreds of millions of dollars to build large-capacity centers with four or five treatment rooms. Statistically, those centers should have been inundated with patients, considering how many people would benefit from proton therapy. That vision proved not to be wrong, but to be premature. Expansion has not proceeded at the anticipated rate. High operating costs and debt service took their toll. Subsequently, one- or two-treatment- room facilities replaced the larger model. None of the smaller centers have experienced financial difficulty.

Muckraking journalists have written negative articles claiming the proton industry is littered with failures. That is not an accurate image. Nor is their claim that hospitals were involved in a medical arms race to gain prestige. The bankruptcies and reorganizations have been at centers, which were developed by only two entities, Advanced Particle Therapy (APT) and ProCure. They were the pioneers. There was no previous model for them to follow.

Cost represents a significant barrier to the availability of proton therapy. Yet, given the technology, much of the cost can't be avoided. The numbers are scary. Early on, large centers had price tags in excess of $200 million. Perhaps developers saw the potential for big profits, but ultimately, that's not what happened.

Take, for example, Advanced Particle Therapy LLC of San Diego (APT). They developed four centers at costs well over $200 million each. The one planned for Dallas went into bankruptcy when major investor oil billionaire Kelcy Warren claimed his $20 million was redirected for other projects and management fees. That center will never be built. Another of their centers at Emory University in Atlanta parted ways with APT and was eventually rescued by Provident, a company in Baton Rouge, Louisiana reorganized with an astronomical debt load of more than $350 million. I don't see how that can possibly work out, even if some of the payments have been deferred to future years when they assume the profitability will have increased.

The first APT project, in San Diego, after three years of operating in the red, went bankrupt in 2017. Scripps had a stellar record of excellent treatment but the cost of leasing the proton center from the developers proved to be too much to handle. A group of doctors calling themselves Proton Doctors Professional Corporation has taken over operation, giving some of the previous creditors ownership in the center. See their listing at the end of the book under California.

Their problems may not be over, however. A law firm specializing in securities fraud, Israels & Neuman, PLC, is soliciting investors who lost money with the developer. During bankruptcy proceedings, the investors blamed Scripps for mismanagement. Scripps said they were strapped by excessive rent and fees. I saw this on the law firm's website (http://www.israelsneuman.com/alert-california-proton-treatment-center-llc/):

Moreover, investors who invested money with the California Proton Treatment Center are likely to face substantial losses with their investment. When securities brokerage firms recommend investments to investors, they have a duty to ensure that the investment is suitable for the investor. The brokerage firm must also perform reasonable research (or due diligence) on the company, so that the firm can adequately disclose the risks of investing in such company. Some brokerage firms who sold investments in the California Proton Treatment Center may not have done the proper due diligence and therefore may not have disclosed all the relevant risks of investing in the proton center.

The brokers who sold the bonds (WFG Investments and Cravens Wealth Advisors, both of Dallas, Texas) may be subject to legal action. What a mess.

The fourth APT center, in Maryland, hasn't gone bankrupt, but recently underwent a financial reorganization. They seem to be doing well.

A further issue for proton centers pertains to over optimistic predictions. The developers of proton centers must get financing, often issuing bonds. For that, they provide a budget and a prospectus predicting future business volume. Since the technology is now applicable to 80% of all cancers, and considering how few centers there are, it would seem that they all should be swamped. And so they make optimistic predictions, which prove true for some cases but not for others. The University of Pennsylvania has been a big success, operating from 7 a.m. to 10 p.m. and is building a second center in New Jersey.

What will be the demand for proton therapy? Some 1,735,350 were diagnosed with cancer in 2018 with 609,640 deaths. If my assumption is correct that 80% of all cancers can be treated with proton therapy which computes to 1,388,280 cases. That's not realistic, of course. MEDRays Intell Proton Therapy World Report says less than 2% of cancer patients are currently treated with proton therapy. That comes to about 34,000 people. In the United States, there are fewer than one hundred treatment rooms for proton therapy, with sixty more in Europe and eighty in Asia. There is one proton therapy room for every sixty-seven X-ray rooms.

By 2030, MEDRays predicts there will be up to 650 treatment rooms worldwide, treating more than 300,000 patients. Yet by my count, the current centers operating in the United States treat about 30,000 people a year. While predicting this huge increase in capability and demand, MEdRays actually shows a slowing of development for 2020. Does that make any sense?

As we will see in the chapter about the future (P.***) , equipment is getting smaller and less expensive, as with any technology, which will make it more accessible to smaller medical centers. So it's easy to see why proton therapy centers justify optimistic predictions. If only these predictions would come true!

To get plenty of business, new proton centers must partner with healthcare institutions in the region, advertise widely, and make themselves visible. One of the best in this regard is the proton center in Irving, Texas, near Dallas. I find their ads on the internet and when taking Southwest Airlines through Love Field in Dallas I have seen large electronic billboards for their services. I also found ads in Southwest's airline magazine.

Provision, where I was treated, announced plans to build a center in New Orleans, but then withdrew after they couldn't find the right local partners. The proton center they are building in Orlando has run into similar delays. A planned center in Baton Rouge had a setback when a co-sponsor got cold feet.

A survey by IBA found the following barriers to the advance of proton therapy.

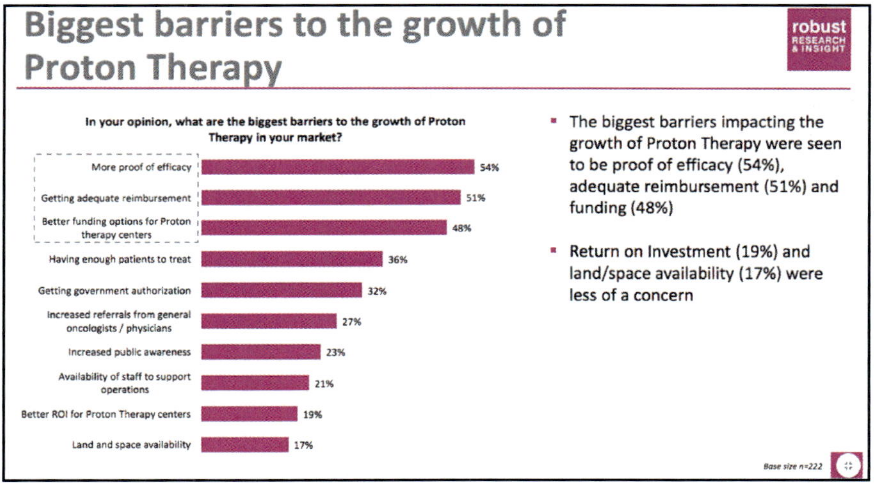

Here are what I think are the main obstacles.

1. Referrals from the medical community have not been forthcoming. They are more likely to resist proton therapy as a threat to their business and pocketbook.

2. It takes decades, sometimes, before new technologies are fully embraced. Proton therapy's time will come. Fortunately, it is available today, even if under less than ideal circumstances.

3. Double blind trials and peer reviews are the traditional means of gaining recognition. Most of the studies we see today equivocate the conclusions, saying proton therapy *may* get better results or has *promise* for the future. Some critics will wait for a

larger body of scientific evidence before they embrace proton therapy for what it is.

4. Misinformation, conflicting studies, and downright distortion deter not only cancer patients, many hospitals themselves are unsure about whether proton therapy is worth the cost of development. No one wants to invest a hundred million dollars into something dubious.

I have concluded that protons must go public, reaching the potential client directly instead of waiting for them to be referred by the medical establishment. Think of the pharmaceutical industry and its many advertisements for prescription drugs. "Ask your doctor if Xefogramabud is right for you. The side effects are . . . . horrifying." If protons advertise, at least they can honestly say there are few side effects.

Negative balance sheets can be tolerated for a while, but eventually the numbers must work: affordable for the patient, profitable for the proton center, covered by Medicare or other insurance, and cost-effective when compared to alternatives. Yet, despite my affinity for numbers, I can't make them work. Provision, for example, cost one hundred and thirty million dollars to build, has a huge building and sophisticated equipment to maintain, and requires a staff of at least sixty. They treated about 600 people the year I was there. How can six hundred patients per year generate enough income to pay for this and still be profitable? Well, they can't. In 2017, Provision lost $1.7 million. They have profits from other areas in their company, so that's not a problem.

As this 2020 edition goes to press, a huge threat to proton therapy is being proposed by the Centers for Medicare and Medicaid Services (CMS). Encouraged by the x-ray community, Medicare is proposing to reimburse all forms of radiation at the same rate. That means proton therapy would receive only the amount typically paid for x-rays, which is at least 50% less. This will not only delay the progress of proton therapy, it might throw some of the centers into serious financial difficulty. To determine the average cost, Medicare looked at radiation claims over a period of 2017-2019. However, only 0.7% of these claims were for proton therapy. The fact is, they can't have a single rate. It you raised the rate to accommodate proton therapy, then you would pay too much for x-rays.

I spent two months investigating how this draconian regulation came into being. For details, see my extensive blog at www.proton-beam-therapy.com/blog.CMS.html. These are the points I made:

1. The proposed rule represents an attack on proton therapy by proponents of x-rays, hijacking CMS procedures for their own purposes.
2. CMS based its policy on outdated studies and sources that do not accurately reflect the true picture and performance of proton therapy.
3. The amount of proof demanded of proton therapy is unreasonable, excessive, and probably unethical.
4. The proposed rule would impede the development of proton therapy, which promises to be the cancer treatment of the future.
5. The physics and technologies of x-rays and proton therapy are substantially different, producing differing results. To suggest an equivalency of value and payment is unsupportable.
6. The CMS policy is based on studies and input from people who have no direct experience with proton therapy. Their understanding is theoretical and their actions uncaring.
7. Thwarting proton therapy will deny the general public of an effective choice in fighting cancer, thereby reducing the quality of available care.
8. The rule needs more time to be considered properly, without a hasty rush to judgment.

If you are reading this book, you are already being more proactive than most patients who just acquiesce without questioning or becoming involved. I don't know what that number is, the percentage of people who take control of their own treatment options. I suspect the internet makes research much easier. In today's medical arena, I think being proactive is necessary. Your life and/or livelihood could hang in the balance. That's what it takes to discover proton therapy for yourself. Congratulations for being a part of that privileged group and taking the first step.

9
HISTORY

How did we get to this point with proton therapy? Three people stand out for their contributions in the development of proton therapy. The first is William Henry Bragg, professor of physics and mathematics at Adelaide University in Australia from 1896 to 1909. He discovered the phenomenon of protons stopping amid a burst of energy. When the energy release is graphed, there is a slow incline and then all of a sudden a spike that goes almost straight up and then back down to nothing. We call this spike the Bragg's Peak, after this gentleman. Little could he have imagined proton therapy today.

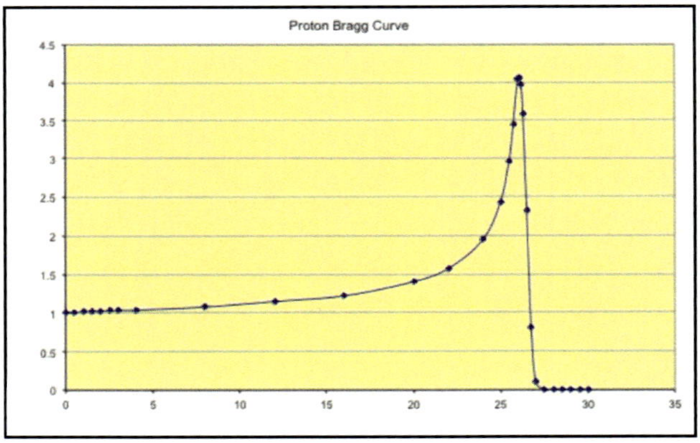

For a technical discussion of the Bragg's Peak, see this link to Brookhaven National Laboratory: https://www.bnl.gov/nsrl/userguide/bragg-curves-and-peaks.php. They describe the above graph.

As we have seen, one or more protons are present in the nucleus of every atom. Each element has a unique number of protons which determine its atomic number and place in the periodic table of elements. Hydrogen, which provides the protons for proton therapy, has a single proton in each atom. Thus, it's number is one on the chart (far left, top).

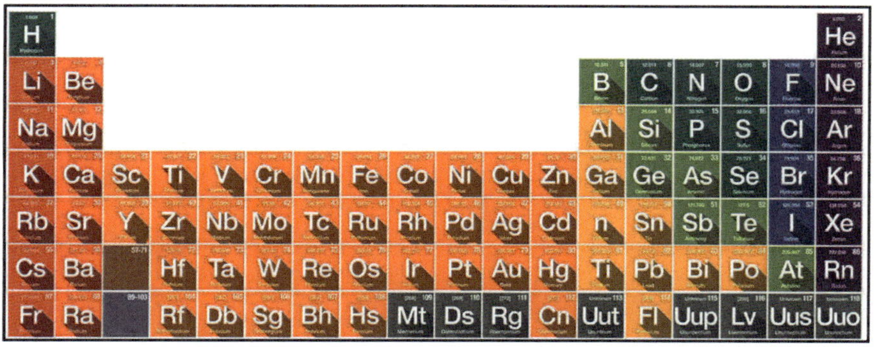

The periodic table of elements, showing hydrogen (H) as number one. Helium (He) is number two, with two protons.

The word proton is Greek for "first," a name coined by Ernest Rutherford in 1920. That makes sense since they use the first element to derive the protons. (A company in England is currently developing five proton therapy centers which will incorporate Rutherford in their names, in recognition of this association.)

Our account then jumps to World War II. In 1943, a young physicist named Robert Rathbun Wilson joined the efforts in Los Alamos, New Mexico for the ultra secret Manhattan Project to develop a nuclear weapon. Still in his twenties, he was the youngest group leader, using a cyclotron shipped to Los Alamos from Harvard University to study measurements of the neutron cross section of plutonium.

After Germany had surrendered, Wilson felt research should stop, but it continued until two nuclear bombs devastated Japan. Thereafter, Wilson lobbied for international control of nuclear weapons. He joined a group of scientists and physicists in developing more powerful particle accelerators for the application of nuclear medicine for diagnostic and medical purposes. Wilson believed protons could be used to reach previously untreatable tumors within the body. He helped design a new 150 MeV cyclotron for Harvard, where he became an associate professor.

In 1946, Wilson published a seminal paper, "Radiological

Use of Fast Protons," which founded proton therapy. I have read the paper, which is just a few pages long. The key, in my mind, is that he understood so intimately the working of cyclotrons and accelerated charged particles.

In 1954, the first human was treated with proton beams at the Lawrence Berkeley Laboratory in California. Eight years later, proton treatments began at the Harvard Cyclotron Laboratory, followed in the mid-1970s by treatments for ocular cancers and larger tumors. It was at Harvard that much of the physics and procedures used for proton therapy were formulated. I find this rather ironic as today, some of the criticism of proton therapy comes from doctors associated with Harvard, and even working in the proton therapy center at Mass General Hospital. Experimentation with the medical uses of protons continued there for decades, treating 9,116 patients before the cyclotron was shut down in 2002 (and subsequently replaced with the current proton center).

After a stint at Cornell, Wilson was chosen to be the director of the Fermi National Accelerator Laboratory (named after Enrico Fermi) usually called Fermilab, where he had a direct role in the design of its buildings and campus. He had studied art and peppered the grounds with his own sculptures. His most lasting contribution was the development of their laboratory building, which he didn't want to look like a drab government structure.

He found his inspiration in Gothic cathedrals, especially the one in Beauvais, France, the tallest exemplar. And so he designed a tall, elegant building with a soaring atrium in the middle. In 1980, the building was renamed Robert Rathbun Wilson Hall in his honor. Curiously, he also introduced a herd of Buffalo that still roam the grounds. See their website: http://www.fnal.gov/pub/about/index.html.

Wilson resigned as director of Fermilab in 1978 to protest what he felt was inadequate funding and support from the federal government. In the initial building stage, he was allotted two hundred fifty million dollars. Construction came in on time and under budget.

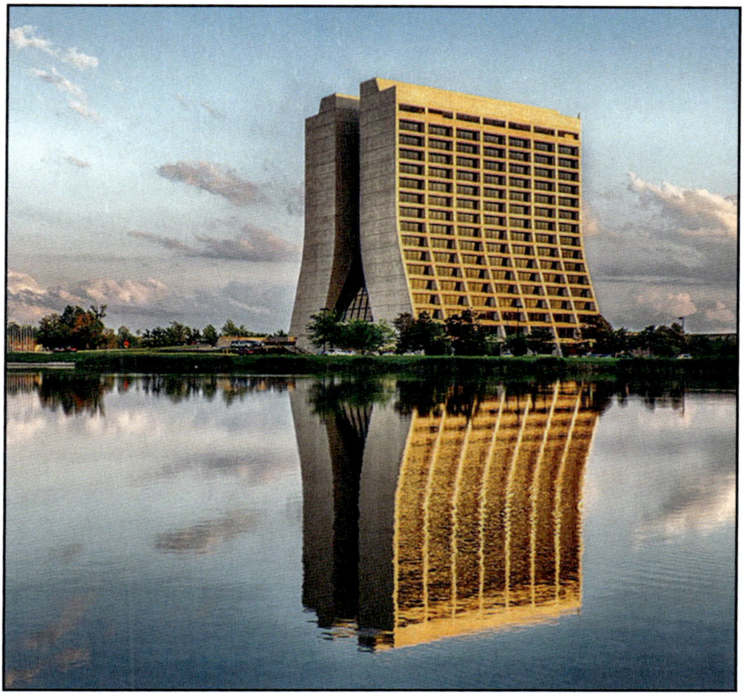

The building Wilson helped design.

Meanwhile, relevant technologies continued to advance, including accelerators, magnetically scanned beams, treatment planning systems, computed tomographic (CT) imaging, and magnetic resonance imaging (MRI).

Proton therapy could be performed only where there were accelerators, whether cyclotrons or synchrotrons. The world's first hospital-based proton therapy center was a low-energy cyclotron equipped centre for ocular tumors at the Clatterbridge Centre for Oncology in the United Kingdom, opened in 1989.

A few years before that date, at Loma Linda University in California, the medical center was seeking someone to build a proton synchrotron (an accelerator that works a little differently from a cyclotron in how it accelerates protons) and beam transport system. The University dedicated a million and a half dollars to the project. That act of vision, in my mind, was the single most important step in the development of proton beam therapy as an accessible treatment.

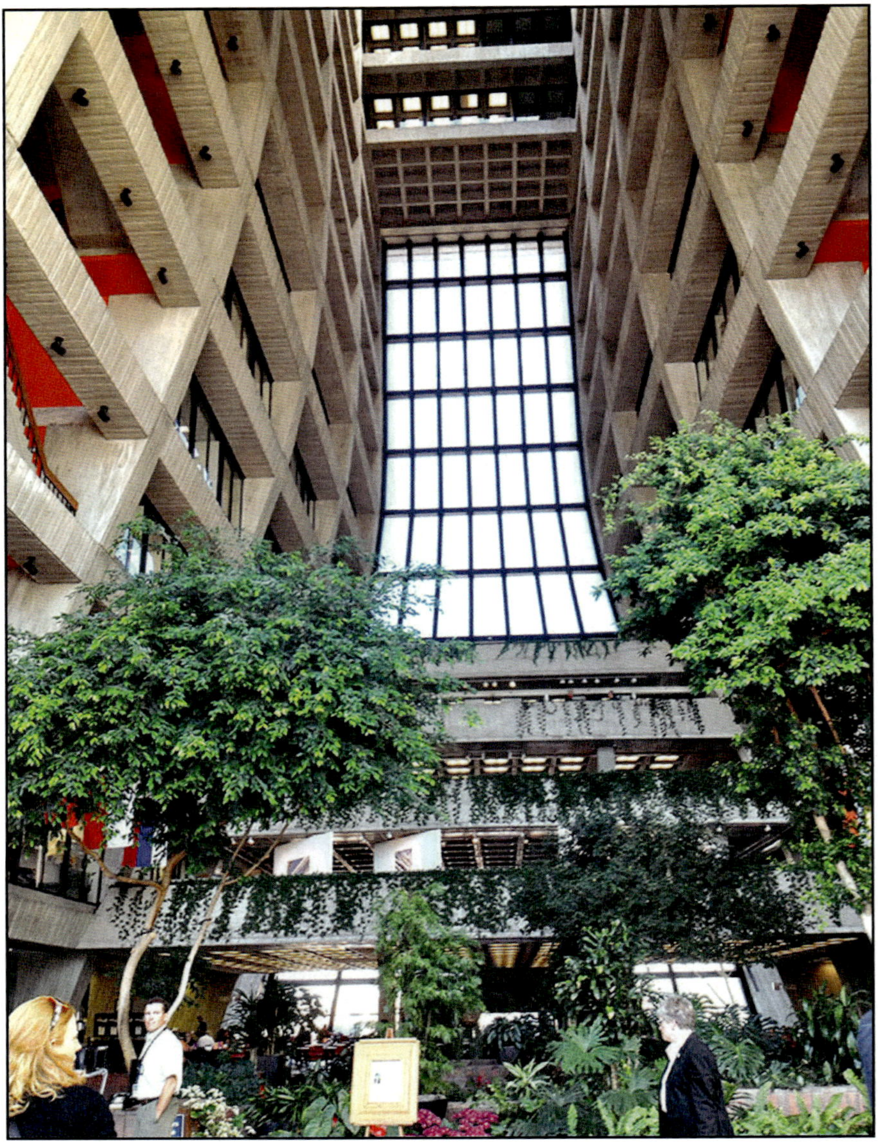

The inside of Wilson's laboratory building.

After several companies had turned down the challenge, Loma Linda contacted Fermilab the same facility founded by

Robert Wilson. Fermilab agreed to build the system, for which the cost and installation became so high the United States government finally came to the rescue with twenty-five million additional dollars. What are the chances something like that would happen today?

This effort was promoted and overseen by our third proton pioneer, Dr. James M. Slater, MD, a researcher in the Loma Linda radiation department. In 1990 the first patient was treated at what was the first hospital-based proton treatment center with equipment powerful enough to penetrate the body and treat cancer. In 1994 the second and third gantries became operational. In 2007 Loma Linda renamed the center the James M. Slater, MD, Proton Treatment and Research Center, currently headed by his son, Jerry D. Slater, MD. In its twenty-nine plus years it has treated more than twenty-one thousand cancer patients encompassing twenty different types of cancer. Loma Linda University led the way for the development of other centers.

It took thirteen years before the next full proton therapy center opened, at Mass General Hospital in 2003 (replacing their old cyclotron). Three years later the third center opened at MD Anderson in Houston, Texas followed shortly by the fourth at the Proton Therapy Institute in Jacksonville, Florida a nonprofit organization affiliated with the University of Florida College of Medicine and the University of Florida Shands Cancer Center.

It took almost two decades before the sixth opened. In the ensuing years, twenty-six more centers have opened, with sixteen more in the planning or building stages. I keep a complete current list on my website, www.proton-therapy-centers.com.

10
THE FUTURE

While I present proton therapy as fighting resistance from the medical community, don't think for a moment that it's in any way "alternative." This new competition with X-rays is coming firmly from within the establishment. At Provision CARES Proton Therapy Center in Knoxville, Tennessee where I was treated, the proton center is part of a much larger practice that includes chemotherapy, X-rays, and other mainstream modalities. They do trials for Big Pharma. The doctors do not hesitate to prescribe drugs. I don't get along well with medicine for profit, but I surely do like protons.

Provision is unique in that they formed a sister company, ProNova, to manufacture proton therapy equipment. They are on the leading edge of pencil beam scanning and superconducting technology. My wife Linda and I toured their very impressive facility.

Superconducting magnets must be powerful to bend the proton beam and control its direction. At ProNova workers wind the magnets on-site and then encase them in highly insulated containers in which they lower the temperature to three degrees Kelvin (about 450 degrees below zero Fahrenheit). The outer shell remains at room temperature. The low temperature effectively reduces electrical resistance to almost nil. Otherwise, the current would cause heat, need to be massive, and would take enormous amounts of electricity to cool.

ProNova's superconducting magnets draw four watts! Four! (Compare to a 60-watt light bulb.) Cyclotrons typically require outrageous amounts of electricity, with electrical bills approaching a million dollars a year. Now, superconducting cyclotrons are under development. They will be smaller, easier to transport, and far more efficient. Maybe someday it will be as ubiquitous as X-rays.

Because of my renewed interest in protons, I have taken to reading about physics. I recently read several books about the Large Hadron Collider (LHC), an amazing underground facility straddling the border of Switzerland and France. It's purpose is to speed up protons and crash them together to examine the smallest parts of atoms and how the work. The LHC is a tunnel seventeen miles in circumference.

Just as with proton therapy, to control the protons they need strong magnets. Accordingly, they have 1,232 dipole superconducting magnets, each more than thirty feet long and weighing thirty-five tons. It took more than twenty years to build the LHC at a cost of nine billion dollars, shared by several countries. I mention it here to make my point of the complex equipment needed in a much smaller scale for proton therapy.

Imaging is an important part of proton therapy. You must be able to accurately identify and locate the tumor. Hence the MRI, CT scans, and X-rays that are part of treatment. New technology often includes cone beam imaging built right into the proton equipment.

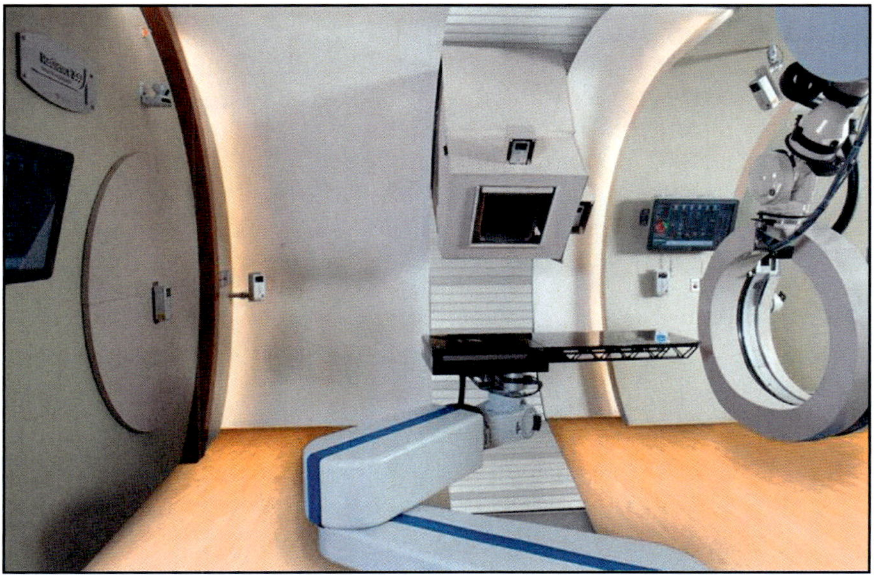

The Radiance 330 system by ProTom.

ProTom International is developing proton tomography, a far more accurate type of imaging that uses protons instead of X-rays. It calls for 350 Mev of energy, which requires a synchrotron instead of a cyclotron. (A cyclotron has a fixed energy output, whereas synchrotrons are adjustable.) Other companies, including Mevion, are also looking into proton imaging.

The first ProTom installation is being completed at Mass General Hospital in Boston even as I write this. It has no huge gantry, requiring a much smaller area and less shielding. So, it's being built into an existing space formerly occupied by two LINAC machines (X-rays). This reduces the cost to a very manageable level that would be suitable for many existing facilities. They seem to be the only company targeting this market.

Other companies are constantly upgrading their technology, as well. For example, the following press release from IBA summarizes the current state of their equipment.

The Proteus®PLUS . . . is configured with two gantry treatment rooms equipped with IBA's pencil beam scanning (PBS) and Cone Beam Computed Tomography (CBCT) large field of view image guidance. These technologies improve the precision of treatment and enable adaptive treatment. The center also benefits from the most advanced room matching available, enabling maximum flexibility of room scheduling and allowing for a minimum 30% reduction in commissioning time therefore giving maximum flexibility for patient treatment. Rooms are also supplied with IBA's wireless hand pendant, the only wireless patient remote control in the radiation therapy industry as well as a new generation, high accuracy and precision Patient Positioning System.

(IBA has an interesting website at https://iba-worldwide.com/proton-therapy.)

Disclosure: I own some IBA stock. To be honest, it hasn't done that well (it's down about 35%).

Mevion has developed a single-room configuration which it believes will be the most in demand. In their description, they make a little dig, saying none of the centers with their equipment have gone bankrupt.

Several centers that have the earlier S250 model from

Mevion are expanding to get the newer version with Hyperscan pencil beam scanning capability. This includes the proton center in Saint Louis, Missouri. In their promotional videos, they make two claims to being unique. First, they have the fastest switching between layers. Secondly, they have introduced a multi-leaf collimator (MLC) to shape the proton beams laterally. The MLC technology has long been used with X-rays. Adding it to the proton arsenal can help to improve its accuracy by shaping the spots as shown below.

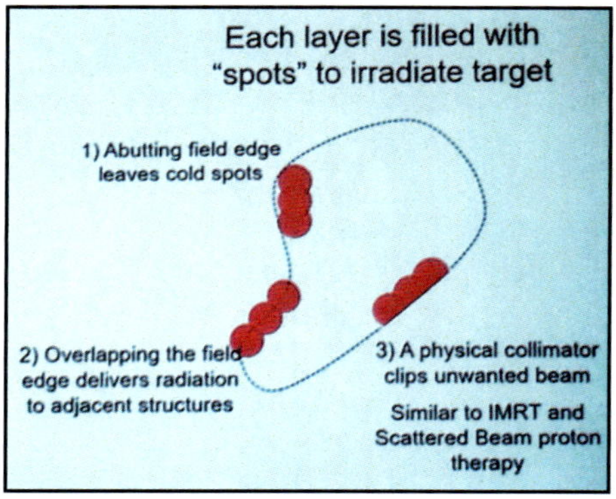

My requested permission to use a graph on Mevion's website was turned down, saying:

There are considerable regulations about how we directly promote or endorse the clinical efficacy of proton therapy. We don't feel comfortable with the tacit endorsement to this use without much closer regulatory review. Thank you for considering us for your book.

I appreciate their principled stand. They would likely think that I have far over-sold proton therapy in this book and made unproven claims as to its efficacy. That's why I like the proton center in Prague. They don't qualify their claims with "may" or "sometimes." They just tell it as they see it. I'm doing the same thing. I'm writing from a patient's point of view, without "considerable regulations" to restrict me.

Varian also made a very principled statement in a press release which I quote here at length:

Statements in this press release regarding future business, plans, objectives, expectations and other similar matters; market acceptance of products or technology for proton therapy; timing and ability to achieve certain results; and any statements using the terms "enables," "offers," "can," "feasible," and "will," are forward-looking statements that involve risks and uncertainties that could cause actual results to differ materially from those anticipated.

These risks and uncertainties include demand for the company's proton therapy products; the company's ability to develop and commercialize new proton therapy products; the company's ability to meet regulatory regulations or procedures; the company's ability to protect the company's intellectual property; and the other risks listed from time to time in the company's filings with the Securities and Exchange Commission, which by this reference are incorporated herein.

These forward-looking statements represent the Company's judgment as of the date of this press release. The Company assumes no obligation to update or revise these forward-looking statements because of new information, future events, or otherwise.

This kind of caution is called due diligence, which is essential in financial dealings. I acknowledge them for the stance they are taking.

Several companies have announced plans to build more proton centers. Provision opened its second center near Memphis, Tennessee and has others planned for Kansas City and Orlando. I found the following in a news release from Providence, a company developing a proton center in Birmingham, Alabama.

Providence Proton Therapy was formed to develop proton therapy cancer treatment centers where they are currently not available, thereby helping cancer patients and local communities. Our goal is to create ten proton therapy centers throughout the United States. Our initial concentration is within the Southeast. Our purpose and desired outcome is unique in terms of developing proton therapy centers in that we are attempting to custom design the structure of each center and the relationship

with a local strategic partner to uniquely fit the needs of the strategic partner and community. In other words, we do not take a "cookie- cutter" or "one size fits all" approach.
(See http://providenceprotontherapy.com/.)

Pardon me for being a bit amused by their assumptions. They want to put proton centers where there aren't any, yet another one is being planned for Birmingham by a different company. And "cookie cutter?" Really? Is there a company just stamping out proton centers? Who?

Another similarly named company, Provident, which took over the difficult situation at Emory University in Atlanta, plans another three centers, one of which will be in Baton Rouge.

In an article called "Three Ways to Make Proton Therapy Affordable," authors Thomas R. Bortfeld and Jay S. Loeffler from suggest these areas for improvement:

1. Shrink accelerators. They are doing this at Mass General with their new ProTom International installation.

2. Sharpen beams. This refers to pencil beam scanning, as preferred over double-scattering. They make this point: "(proton) therapy is not like a pill: its success depends on how it is delivered. It has more room for improvement than other, more-established radiation treatments, such as X-rays."

3. Broaden healthcare coverage. This is indeed essential. In their article, they make a very concise case for protons, which I quote below.

If cost was not an issue, proton therapy would be the treatment of choice for most patients with localized tumours. Protons can be targeted more precisely than X-rays, so the tissues around the tumour receive two to three times less radiation. This lowers the chance of causing secondary tumours or impairing white blood cells and the immune system. High doses of protons can be delivered safely to hard-to-treat tumours: for instance, those at the base of the skull or in the liver. Such accuracy is crucial when treating cancers in children.

From the same article:

Three developments that have emerged in the past three years hold promise. Narrow 'pencil' beams that paint the radiation dose precisely onto a tumour reduce the need to treat patients from many angles. Rapid imaging methods can detect tiny changes in the patient's position, so that the beam can be shifted. And advanced 'soft robotics' built using malleable outer materials will soon allow patients to be positioned quickly and comfortably using robotic hands.
(See: https://www.nature.com/news/three-ways-to-make-proton-therapy-affordable-1.22660)

IBA conducted a survey to find how people see the future of proton therapy. The chart below shows their results.

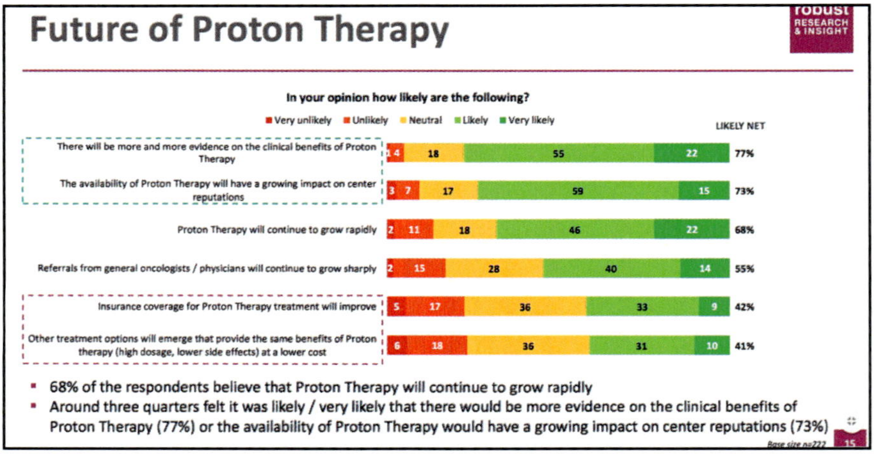

Results from a survey conducted by IBA.

Where will these new centers find staff? Greg Sonnenfeld, director of Shreveport's Willis-Knighton Cancer Center, has said recruiting and retaining specialists well versed in the technology have been a struggle. There has been frequent moving from one center to another. For example, my doctor at Provision, Mario Fagundes, a leader in the field, left in the middle of my stay to go to the new center in Miami (closer to family and his native Brazil). The proton center in Dallas enticed Dr. Andrew K. Lee, a leading proton therapy expert and one of the founders of proton therapy at MD Anderson to become their Medical Director. He was the first physician to treat patients with pencil beam scanning and pioneered the use of fiducial markers. I can see how he might be attracted to a new center with the latest technology.

As more and more centers open it won't work to simply try to snipe experts from other centers. For that reason, Provision has an extensive training program. Then, much like a sous chef at a fine restaurant moving on to open his or her own restaurant after they get some experience, proton workers go into the market place to find new more lucrative opportunities.

The University of Florida addresses this need. All the staff at the Proton Therapy Institute are faculty members at the university, where they train the next generation of proton therapy workers. If I were a young doctor or radiology technician, I would definitely become involved with proton therapy, an exciting field with great job security.

The equipment manufacturer Varian and the University of Pennsylvania Proton Therapy Center have joined to provide a 40-week training program in all aspects of proton therapy, combined with on-site internships. They offer to give their training at other proton centers, as well. So, some steps are being taken to meet the need.

Another possibility is for personnel experienced with X-rays to switch to protons. Since both involve radiation, many procedures are the same. If X-ray practitioners are feeling threatened by proton therapy, why not jump ship? As you can gather from this chapter, proton therapy is where the action is right now. Why not join the crowd?

The height of development for proton therapy seemed to be about 2015 and 2016. Then, some of the larger centers began to develop financial difficulties, resulting in some restructuring or bankruptcies. That seemed to put a brake on predictions for the future.

One source had predicted a need for 300 treatment centers within a decade, almost ten times what we have now. Then, they reduced their estimate by 20%, which is still no slouch.

Now, the trend is strongly toward one-room developments, with a single gantry. Some systems have the gantry built right into the treatment room facility, whereas others have a separate cyclotron that can be upgraded in the future to accommodate several more treatment rooms.

In late December, 2019, on a website called News Cast Report, I found a new seven-year prediction that is very favorable. There are a number of companies that do research in various fields and then sell their data. That is the case here, as well, with data amasses by a company called Data Bridge.

Their chart had a rather suspicious uniform consistency to it. I suspect they took the first year and the last year and just averaged out all of the years in between. Nevertheless, it is heartening to see this prediction that by 2026 the market will more than triple. Here is my interpretation of their data.

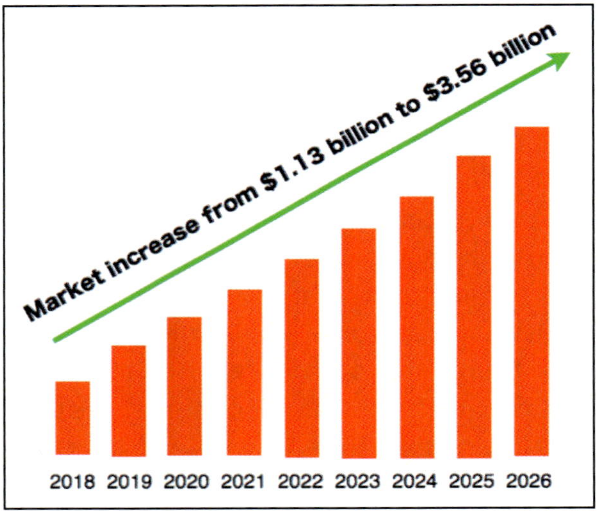

We currently have thirty-five centers open in the United States. We could probably almost double the number of patients treated if all centers operated at full capacity. But to triple the market for proton therapy, we are going to need far more than the fifteen centers I have listed under "planned or under construction" (see p.

121). That means we ought to be seeing many more announcements for new centers.

If undue criticism were lessened, Medicare and other insurance issues resolved in a favorable way, and costs lowered, the development of proton therapy will soar. Who will be the beneficiaries? All of us cancer patients.

11
MY EXPERIENCE

My first book, *Prostate Cancer Best Treatment: Proton Beam Therapy*, describes in considerable detail my personal cancer and proton therapy journeys. Here, I give a more succinct summary. For more information, see my first book.

It never occurred to me to be watching the health of my prostate. For some unexplainable reason, neither did my family doctor. PSA, prostate specific antigen, can be determined through a blood test. It should be very low. If it starts climbing, men often engage in "watchful waiting." Once it climbs over 4.0, action is usually taken to discover the cause. Other factors can cause the PSA to rise, but once they are ruled out, cancer is the most likely probability.

My PSA continued to rise with little notice. My routine blood tests had several categories that said "high," most of which I didn't understand. So I depended on my healthy lifestyle and diet. Fortunately, in 2016 I changed doctors. He saw my PSA of 12.0 and sounded the alarm. By the time we ruled out noncancerous possibilities, the PSA had climbed to 16.0.

Doing my research, I geared up for the latest technology for scans and targeted biopsy, but my urologist would have none of it. He did the old-fashioned twelve-core pattern biopsy that he has used for thirty years. Even then, seven of the cores showed positive for cancer.

Prostate caner, I found, is very common. There is an adage that says "many more men die *with* prostate cancer than *of* it." Some don't even know they have cancer. Slow-moving cancer can be watched for years before needing treatment, if ever. The exception is when the PSA jumps rapidly. Mine did, doubling twice in two years (3 to 6, then 6 to 12), indicating a more aggressive strain of cancer. Given how long I had waited, I was astoundingly fortunate.

My Gleason score (4+3=7) gave me a grade of intermediate cancer. An MRI showed no spread of the cancer outside the organ itself. A bone scan showed no sign of cancer. My urologist told me to have surgery, although I'm a bit old for that. Since I'm in good shape, he assured me I would likely recover quickly. He called it the gold standard in prostate cancer treatment. He was wrong. Very wrong. Most surveys show that surgery has the worst result, and is least preferred by patients.

I found *An ABC of Prostate Cancer in 2015: My Journey Over 4 Continents to Find the Best Cure*, by Alan G. Lawrenson, a medical researcher in Australia. He covers all the options in great detail. Then, he decided on proton therapy. I figured he knows a lot more than I do; I should pay attention. Since his insurance didn't cover it, he chose to go to South Korea for treatment. When I found that my United Healthcare insurance wouldn't cover proton therapy, I, too, considered going abroad, perhaps to Prague.

On a Friday, I sent out an email to a dozen proton therapy centers, asking what their out-of-pocket cost would be. On Saturday, I received by overnight mail a package from the Texas Center for Proton Therapy near Dallas. Very impressive. They understood my sense of urgency. First thing Monday morning, I got a call from Samantha at Provision CARES Proton Therapy Center in Knoxville, Tennessee. She told me the cost ($93,000) and then asked whether I'm on Medicare. That led to the discovery of the registry that I have already described, and the subsequent two-month-long stay in Knoxville.

Interestingly, two other proton centers are on the same registry. One is Ackerman Cancer Center in Jacksonville, Florida and the other is Texas Center for Proton Therapy. If I had a chance to do it over, I would likely go to Dallas. Searching for other registries at other centers has proved to be difficult. I suggest that the reader make that inquiry of any proton center under consideration. Some registries are voluntary and offer no reimbursement.

Please note the difference between a registry and a randomized trial. A registry tracks the results of a certain technology, in this case proton therapy, over the long term. A randomized trial tests two different treatments, for which each group is randomly selected. My wife's cousin Larry was diagnosed with prostate cancer. He was considering surgery until I sent him a copy of my book. When his doctor asked whether he would be in a trial, he said no. Preferring proton therapy, Larry didn't want to chance that he would be assigned X-rays. He received proton therapy at Mass General in Boson which was paid by his government insurance (he's a retired postal worker). Today he's just fine.

So Linda and I went to Knoxville for two months. Our little cottage was cute as a button, only three miles from the proton center, requiring no highways or major roads en route. We were half a mile from Whole Foods and just a few blocks from one of the longest commercial streets, chock a block with stores, shopping centers, and restaurants. Further, the cost was very reasonable.

When I write about my cancer journey, I should say our cancer journey, as my wife Linda was with me every step of the way. Together, besides going to the proton center for treatment, we also worked out at the fitness center, took walks every morning, went shopping for groceries, and enjoyed exploring Knoxville.

The time seemed to go slowly. I made a big chart and crossed off each treatment. I attended the graduation ceremonies of many other patients, as they took place right in the lobby. Some were very simple, others had a large group of family members attend, and in one case, a church choir sang. Finally, after the last treatment, I had my graduation ceremony, which involves ringing the victory bell.

This poem is written on the bell:

Ring this bell
Three times well
Its toll to clearly say,
My treatment's done
This course is run
And I am on my way!

Like 1,231 patients at Provision before me, I gave a short speech, praising the staff profusely. Linda and I rang the bell together. Then, we raised our fists in celebration.

The date was November 1, 2016. I received a certificate and other items. It took only a few more minutes for us to climb into our already packed car and start our trip back to San Antonio, hitting numerous Cracker Barrels along the way (sometimes just to take a break, drink a coffee, and rock in those chairs along the front porch).

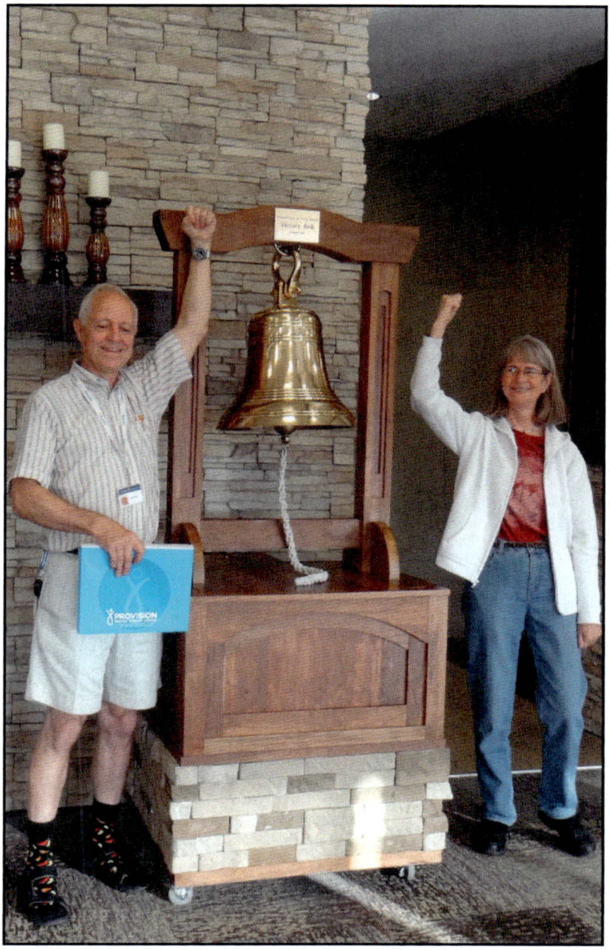

Graduation ceremony

Once home, life immediately returned to normal. I took Flomax for a month or so and then no longer needed it. I had no pain, no restrictions of any kind. I returned to my normal diet and lifestyle. After six months, I had my first checkup, a digital exam and a blood test. My PSA was 1.42. My latest test, in the summer of 2019, was 0.32. I find that I follow exactly the course of post-treatment PSA levels shown in the following graph from the proton therapy center in Prague.

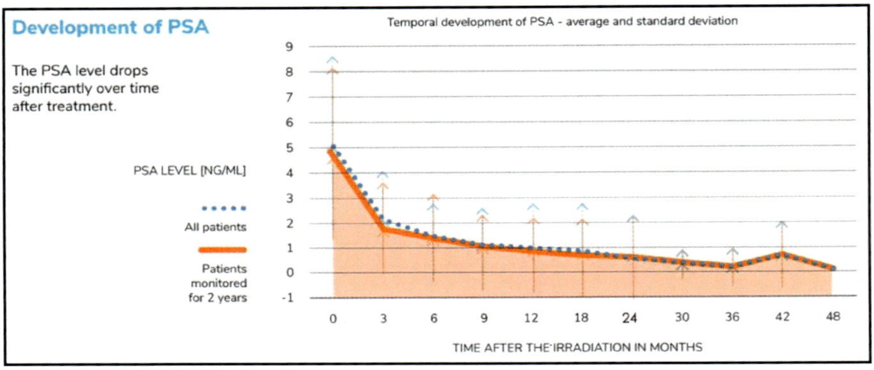

Here, it shows a PSA just above zero at the thirty-six-month stage, which is where I am. It shows a small upward blip for the next exam. We'll see.

For the first couple of years, I also filled out a very long questionnaire every six months that goes into great detail about every aspect of my health, sexual activity, urination, and more. I thought I would be filling out these forms for the rest of my life, but in January, 2019 they were stopped. I don't know why.

Somehow, all this had to be paid for. How much did Medicare actually pay for me to be on the registry? The calculation is very confusing. I received forms in the mail that compared the amount billed to the amount paid. The difference is extreme. The best I can guess, Provision billed a total of almost $300,000 to Medicare and United Healthcare, and (including my copay of $4,500) likely received a little less than a third of that amount. Considering the cash out-of-pocket price they quoted was $93,000, I'm guessing that's about what they received.

When I first arrived in Knoxville, I told myself that I would not work on a book. I would have quality time with Linda and work on my poetry and take it easy. However, I found proton therapy—the experience and the technology—so amazing that I couldn't resist. So I started keeping a journal almost right away, meeting with staff members, physicists, nurses, insurance people, and even the founder of Provision. During treatment, I asked my techs many questions. I knew I had to share this valuable information.

These days, when I give presentations to local groups, almost no one in the audience has heard of proton therapy. My bumper sticker, I LOVE PROTONS, probably puzzles people. Why would I love part of the nucleus of an atom? You, dear reader, could answer that.

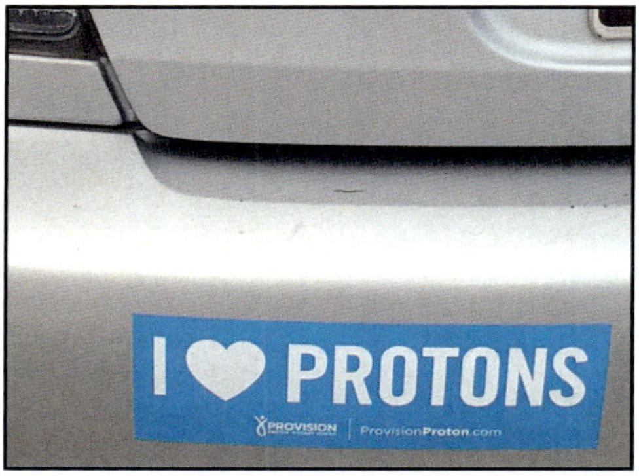

I'm happy to be a proton ambassador, to answer questions, or to come and speak to groups or conferences. I find it unacceptable that the medical community continues to resist proton therapy. I would like to hire giant billboards all around the country encouraging people to learn about proton therapy. One day it should a household word, just as X-rays are today.

My websites continue to grow and hold relevant information. I would like to do more, with social media, videos, and other popular methods of communicating. But I'm a one-pony show. I do this without sponsors or help, at my own expense. You can help in spreading the word. Thanks.

RESOURCES

ProtonTherapyBook.com
Describes my books on proton therapy. Includes scores of full-color photos and illustrations. Free books are available (previous editions).

proton-beam-therapy.com
My proton therapy blog with articles about relevant and timely topics.

proton-therapy-centers.com
An up-to-date listing of proton centers in the United States.

labyrinth-enterprises.com
The original website for my labyrinth-building business (which still has extensive information on that subject). Labyrinth Enterprises LLC now publishes my books.

biomed-research.com
The research division of Provision Healthcare. They sponsor the registry that I am on, which is for all types of cancer treated with protons.

clinicaltrials.gov
List of clinical trials all over the world.

proton-cancer-treatment.com
The English-language website for the proton therapy center in Prague. EU residents are covered. I almost went there for treatment. They have kindly provided me with illustrations I have used in this book.

proton-therapy.org
The website of the National Association for Proton Therapy. They have a ton of information.

proton-therapy-today.com
An online magazine about proton therapy. It doesn't appear to be very up-to-date.

protonbob.com/about-proton-therapy/proton-therapy-myths
On the website of the Brotherhood of the Balloon, this article debunks myths about proton therapy.

allianceforprotontherapy.org
This is a nonprofit organization supported by the proton industry to encourage insurance coverage and report cases, both positive and negative.

protominternational.com
A company specializing in proton tomography, which seems to hold much promise.

ptcog.ch
The Particle Therapy Co-Operative Group, which documents the proton therapy centers in the world. If you are thinking of going abroad for treatment, this would be the place to look.

USE OF INTERNET MATERIAL

Section 107 of the Copyright Act states: "The fair use of a copyrighted work, including such use by reproduction in copies or phonograph records or by any other means specified by that section, for purposes such as criticism, comment, news reporting, teaching (including multiple copies for classroom use), scholarship, or research, is not an infringement of copyright."

I consider this book to be research and educational. I have done my best to attribute photos and illustrations. If I have inadvertently used anything that the owner would like me to remove or properly attribute, please let me know.

PROTON THERAPY CENTERS IN THE UNITED STATES

We now list 35 centers operating in the United States with 15 in planning or construction stages.
PBS = Pencil Beam Scanning
G = Gantry, F = Fixed beam, which includes up to 60 degrees of movement.
Low energy sites are not included.

1. **Alabama, Birmingham**
Proton International
University of Alabama at Birmingham (UAB)
400 20th Street South
Birmingham, AL 35233
www.uabmedicine.org/proton
Tel: 205.934.9999
One gantry, Varian 250si
Open January, 2020

2. **Arizona, Phoenix**
Mayo Clinic Proton Beam Therapy Center
5881 E, Mayo Boulevard, Phoenix, AZ 85054
Tel: 480.369-5200
www.mayoclinic.org/departments-centers/proton-beam-therapy-program/sections/proton-therapy-facilities/gnc-20187682
Opened: 2016
Four gantries
PBS: Yes

3. **California, Loma Linda**
James M. Slater MD Proton Treatment and Research Center
11234 Anderson Street, Loma Linda, CA 92354
Tel: 800.PROTONS (800.776.8667)
www.protons.com

Opened: 1990
Three gantries, one fixed beam
PBS: ?
Treated more than 20,000 patients, pioneered proton therapy

4. **California, San Diego**
California Protons Cancer Therapy Center
9730 Summers Ridge Rd., San Diego, CA 92121
Tel: 858.549.7400
www.californiaprotons.com
Opened: 2014, reorganized 2017
Three gantries, two fixed beam
PBS: 5

5. **Florida, Delray Beach**
South Florida Proton Therapy Institute (SFPTI)
5280 Linton Blvd., Delray Beach, FL 33484
Tel: 561.323.6498
www.sfpti.com/about/
Opened 2018
One Gantry
PBS: Yes

6. **Florida, Jacksonville**
Ackerman Cancer Center
10881 San Jose Boulevard, Jacksonville, FL 32223
Tel: 904.880.5522
www.ackermancancercenter.com/proton-therapy/what-is-proton-therapy/
Opened: 2015
One gantry
PBS: No
First private physician-funded proton center in U.S.
Joined Provision's Medicare registry for proton therapy.

7. **Florida, Jacksonville**
University of Florida Proton Therapy Institute

2015 N. Jefferson Street, Jacksonville, FL 32206
Tel: 904.588.1800
www.floridaproton.org
Opened: 2006
Three gantries, one fixed beam, one new treatment room in 2019
PBS: Yes

8. **Florida, Miami**
Miami Cancer Institute at Baptist Health South
8900 N Kendall Dr, Miami, FL 33176
786.527.8010, 786.596.2000
www.baptisthealth.net/cancer-care/treatments-and-services/radiation-therapies/proton-therapy
Three gantries
PBS: Yes, all
Opened 2018

9. **Florida, Orlando**
The Marjorie and Leonard Williams Center for Proton Therapy, University of Florida Health Center
1400 S. Orange Avenue, Orlando, FL 32806
Tel: 321.841.8650 / 321.841.1869
www.ufhealthcancerorlando.com/centers/proton-therapy-center
Opened: 2016
One partial gantry (Mevion S250), 15,000 sq. ft. facility
PBS: No

10. **Georgia, Atlanta**
Emory Proton Treatment Center
615 Peachtree Street NE, Atlanta GA 30308
707.217.7565
www.winshipcancer.emory.edu/proton-therapy-center
Opened: 2018
4 Gantries, 1 Fixed Beam
PBS: Yes

11. **Illinois, Warrenville**

Northwestern Medicine Chicago Proton Center
4455 Weaver Parkway, Warrenville, IL 60555 (Chicago area)
Tel: 877.887.5807
www.chicagoprotoncenter.com
Opened: 2010
One gantry, three fixed beam
PBS: No

12. **Louisiana, Shreveport**
Willis-Knighton Proton Therapy Center
2600 Kings Highway, Shreveport, LA 71103
Tel: 318.212.8300
www.wkhs.com/Cancer/Cancer-Treatment-Services/Proton-Therapy/Proton-Therapy-Facts.aspx
Opened: 2014
One gantry (IBA ProteusONE)
PBS: Yes

13. **Maryland, Baltimore**
Maryland Proton Treatment Center
850 West Baltimore Street, Baltimore, MD 21201
Tel: 410.369.5200
www.mdproton.com
Opened: 2016
Three gantries, two fixed beams
PBS: Yes
Charges the same for proton therapy as for X-ray radiation.

14. **Massachusetts, Boston**
Francis H. Burr Proton Therapy Center Massachusetts General Hospital
30 Fruit Street
Boston, MA 02114
617.726.0923
Proton Inquiry Line: Tel: 617.724.1680
www.massgeneral.org/radiationoncology/BurrProtonCenter.aspx
Opened: 2003

Two gantries, one fixed beam
2019: New synchrotron-powered system by ProTom coming oline with PBS
PBS: Yes

15. **Michigan, Flint**
Mclaren Proton Therapy Center
4100 Beecher Road, Flint, MI 48532
Tel: 855.697.7684
www.mclaren.org/main/proton-therapy-center
Opened 2019
One ProTom Radiance 330 synchrotron
PBS: Yes

16. **Michigan, Royal Oak**
Proton Therapy Center at Beaumont Hospital Cancer Institute
3601 W. Thirteen Mile Road, Royal Oak, MI 48073
Tel: 248.551.8402
www.beaumont.org/treatments/proton-therapy
Opened July, 2017
One IBA ProteusOne gantry
PBS: Yes

17. **Minnesota, Rochester**
Mayo Clinic Proton Beam Therapy Center
190 Second Street NW, Rochester, MN 55901
Tel: 507.284.2511
www.mayoclinic.org/departments-centers/proton-beam-therapy-program/sections/proton-therapy-facilities/gnc-20187682
Opened: 2015
Four gantries
PBS: Yes
They do many clinical trials.

18. **Missouri, St. Louis**
S. Lee Kling Proton Therapy Center
St. Louis, MO

Tel: 314.286.1222
www.siteman.wustl.edu/treatment/siteman-approach/radiation/proton-beam-therapy/
Opened: 2013
One gantry (Mevion S250) and one S250i with PBS
PBS: Yes

19. **New Jersey, Brunswick**
The Laurie Proton Therapy Center Robert Wood Johnson University Hospital
One Robert Wood Johnson Place, New Brunswick, NJ 08901
Tel: 888.MD.RWJUH
www.rwjuh.edu/proton-therapy/proton-therapy.aspx
Opened: 2015
One gantry
PBS: ?

20. **New Jersey, Somerset**
ProCure Proton Therapy Center
103 Cedar grove Lane, Somerset, NJ 08873
Tel: 877.967.7628
www.procure.com/New-Jersey-Explore
Open: 2012
Four gantries
PBS: Yes

21. **New York, New York**
New York Proton Center
225 E. 126th Street
New York, NY 10035
833.697.7686
www.newyorkprotoncenter.com
2019
5 Gantries
PBS: Yes

22. **Ohio, Cincinnati**
Children's Proton Therapy Center
7777 Yankee Road
Liberty Township, OH 45044
Tel: 877.881.8479, 513.636.2866
www.cincinnatichildrens.org/service/p/proton-therapy
Opened: 2016
Three gantries
PBS: Yes

23. **Ohio, Cleveland**
University Hospital Seidman Cancer Center
11100 Euclid Avenue, Cleveland, OH 44106
Tel:855.318.8390
www.uhhospitals.org/seidman/services/radiation-oncology/our-technology/proton-therapy
Opened: 2016
One gantry
PBS: No

24. **Oklahoma, Oklahoma City**
Oklahoma Proton Center
5901 W. Memorial Road, Oklahoma City, OK 73142
Tel: 888.847.2640
www.OKCproton.com
Opened: 2009, reorganized in 2018
One gantry, three fixed beam
PBS: No

25. **Oklahoma, Oklahoma City**
Stephenson Cancer Center Proton Center at the University of Oklahoma
800 NE 10th Street, Oklahoma City, OK 73104
Tel: 855.750.2273
www.stephensoncancercenter.org/Patients/Clinics-Services/Proton-Therapy

Opened: 2015 / 2019
Clinitron 250TM by Mevion
PBS: Yes

26. **Pennsylvania, Philadelphia**
Roberts Proton Therapy Center
University of Pennsylvania Penn Medicine
3400 Civic Center Boulevard, Philadelphia, PA 19104
Tel: 800.789.7366
www.pennprotontherapy.org
Year opened: 2010
IBA: Four gantries, one fixed beam, one research
PBS: No
Calls itself largest in the world (not)

27. **Tennessee, Franklin (Nashville)**
Provision CARES Proton Therapy Nashville
4588 Carothers Parkway
Franklin, TN 37067
844.726.8884
www.nashvilleproton.com
Opened: 2018
Two gantries, one fixed beam
ProNova equipment

28. **Tennessee, Knoxville**
Provision CARES Proton Therapy Center
6450 Provision Cares Way, Knoxville, TN 37909
Tel: 865.862.1600
www.provisionproton.com
Year opened: 2014
Two gantries one fixed beam (IBA) and
one gantry one fixed beam (ProNova)
PBS: Yes

29. **Tennessee, Memphis**
St. Jude Red Frog Events Proton Therapy Center (Children only)

262 Danny Thomas Place, Memphis, TN 38105
Tel: 866.278.5833
www.stjude.org/treatment/services/radiation-oncology/proton-therapy.html
Opened: 2015
Two gantries, one fixed beam
PBS: Yes
Red Frog Events raised millions for the center, hence the name.

30. **Texas, Houston**
MD Anderson Proton Therapy Center
1840 Old Spanish Trail, Houston, TX 77054
Tel: 866.632.4782
www.mdanderson.org/patients-family/diagnosis-treatment/care-centers-clinics/proton-therapy-center.html
Opened: 2006
Three gantries, one fixed beam
PBS: The first to have it.
Huge expansion planned.

31. **Texas, Irving (Dallas)**
Texas Center for Proton Therapy
1501 West Royal Lane, Irving, TX 75063
Tel: 469.513.5500
www.texascenterforprotontherapy.com
Opened: 2015
Two gantries, one fixed beam
IBA Proteus technology
PBS: Yes

32. **Virginia, Hampton**
Hampton University Proton Therapy Institute
40 Enterprise Parkway, Hampton, VA 23666
Tel: 757.251.6800
www.hamptonproton.org
Opened: 2010
Four gantries, one fixed beam

PBS: No

33. **Washington, Seattle**
SCCA Proton Therapy Center
1570 North 115th Street, Seattle WA 98133
Tel: 877.897.7628
www.sccaprotontherapy.com
Date opened: 2013
One gantry, two fixed beam
PBS: No

34. **Washington, D.C.**
Georgetown Lombardi Comprehensive Cancer Center at Medstar Georgetown University Hospital
3800 Reservoir Road, N.W., Washington DC 20057
Tel: 855.546.2805
www.medstargeorgetown.org/our-services/cancer-care/treatments/proton-beam-therapy/
Date opened: 2018
Gantries: 1 (first Mevion 250Si with pencil beam scanning and Hyperscan imagery) with pencil beam scanning.

35. **Washington, D.C.**
Johns Hopkins National Proton Therapy Center
Sibley Memorial Hospital
5255 Loughboro Road NW,
Washington, DC 20016
Tel: 202.804.3343
www.hopkinsmedicine.org/kimmel_cancer_center/centers/proton-therapy-center/
Date opened: 2019
Three gantries

PROTON CENTERS PLANNED OR UNDER CONSTRUCTION

All are assumed to have Pencil Beam Scanning (PBS)

1. **Alabama, Birmingham**
Providence Proton Center
St. Vincents - Birmingham
1200 Corporate Drive, Suite 470, Birmingham, AL 35242
James Curtis: Tel: 205.451.7839
www.providenceprotontherapy.com/
Opening: Delayed
One gantry, IBA Proteus

2. **Connecticut, Wallingford**
Proton International Proton Therapy Center
932 Northrup Road
Wallingford, CT 06492
One gantry
Opening 2023

3. **Florida, Jacksonville**
Mayo Clinic Proton Therapy Center
Jacksonville, FL
Opening: 2023
Two gantries
This will be the third proton center in Jacksonville

4. **Florida, Miami**
The Sylvester Comprehensive Cancer Center at the University of Miami Miller School of Medicine
1475 NW 12th Ave, Miami, FL 33136
305.699-6417
www.umiamihealth.org/Sylvester
Opening: Mid-2020
Gantries: 1

5. **Florida, Orlando**
Provision CARES Proton Therapy Center, Orlando
15775 New Independence Parkway
Winter Garden, Florida.
Opening: 2022
Two gantries plus one fixed beam (ProNova)

6. **Kansas, Kansas City**
University of Kansas Health System
4000 Cambridge, Kansas City, KS
913.588.1227
www.kansashealthsystem.com
Opening: 2021
One gantry, IBA Proteus One

7. **Kansas, Kansas City**
Provision CARES Cancer Center and Proton Therapy Center
Kansas City, KS
Opening: 2022
Two gantries, one fixed beam
ProNova equipment

8. **Louisiana, Baton Rouge**
Louisiana Proton Care Center
Provident Proton Care, a division of Provident Resource Group
Baton Rouge, LA
Being downsized.

9. **Missouri, St. Louis**
Mercy Hospital
615 New Ballas Road, St. Louis, MO 63141
314.251.6000
One gantry
Opening: 2022

10. **New Jersey, Voorhees Township**
Virtua Voorhees Hospital
100 Bowman Drive, Voorhees Township, NJ 08043
856.247.3000
www.virtua.org/news/proton-therapy-to-south-jersey
In conjunction with Penn Medicine
One gantry, Varian
Opening: 2022

11. **North Carolina, Durham**
Duke University Health System
Durham, NC
Two treatment rooms by ProNova
Open: 2021

12. **Ohio, Columbus**
Ohio State University's James Cancer Hospital and Nationwide Children's Hospital
410 W 10th Avenue
Columbus, Ohio 43210
614.293.8000
Opening: 2022

13. **Pennsylvania, Lancaster**
Lancaster General Health Proton Therapy Center
Lancaster, PA
888.544.4636
One treatment room
Opening: 2021

14. **Utah, Salt Lake City**
Huntsman Cancer Institute
University of Utah
2000 Circle of Hope
Salt Lake City, Utah 84103
(801) 585-0100
www.healthcare.utah.edu/huntsmancancerinstitute/

Opening: late 2020

15. **Virginia, Fairfax**
Center for Advanced Radiation Oncology and Proton Therpy
Inova Schar Cancer Institute
8081 Innovation Park Drive
Fairfax, VA 22031
Tel: 571.472.0606
www.virginiaradiation.com/locations/inova-schar-cancer-institute/
Opening: 2020
Two gantries, IBA ProteusOne with pencil beam scanning and cone beam imaging

FOREIGN PROTON CENTERS OF INTEREST

1. Prague, Czechoslovakia
www.proton-cancer-treatment.com

2. Shanghai, China
shmtppp.com

3. Seoul, Korea
www.nccproton.com

4. Galgenen, Switzerland
www.psi.ch/protontherapy/

5. Apollo Hospitals, in India
Proton therapy center opening in mid-2017.

www.apollohospitals.com/departments/cancer/treatment/radiation-therapy

Also see www.ptcog.ch/index.php/facilities-in-operation for proton centers around the world.

FINAL NOTE

I WELCOME input from readers of this and any other of my books or websites. My preferred method of contact is via email at this address: robert@ProtonTherapyBook.com. My other proton therapy book is *Prostate Cancer Treatment: Proton Therapy*. If you have enjoyed this book, or learned from it, please leave a favorable review on Amazon.

After my wife Ruth Hanna, to whom this book is dedicated, died of breast cancer in 2007, I couldn't imagine ever having another relationship. Six months later, I met Linda. We stayed in touch until I was ready, getting married in May of 2010. Our courtship and love affair were closely tied to cruise ships and transatlantic voyages. I wrote a memoir about our love story called *Cruise of the Heart*: *Memoir of a Transatlantic Voyage*. It describes the cruise industry much like this book does proton beam therapy. You'll find it available in both print and kindle versions on Amazon.

For more than twenty years I've been a full time labyrinth builder, leading me to write some instructional and informational books including the following:

The Labyrinth Revival: A Personal Account
Constructing the Chartres Labyrinth
Constructing Classical Labyrinths
Canvas Labyrinths Construction Manual
Church Labyrinths
Origin, Symbolism and Design of the Chartres Labyrinth

I give the proceeds from these books to Veriditas, a nonprofit organization that supports the use of labyrinths. In my retirement, I have more writing projects planned, about happiness, about aging, and other topics. Thank you for your interest in this book. Please share this information with everyone you know.

Robert Ferré
January 2020

BOOK REVIEW

Saving Ashya by Naghmeh King

In *Saving Ashya*, British author Naghmeh King relates a harrowing tale of what was necessary to get proton therapy for her five-year-old son Ashya King who was diagnosed with a brain tumor. After their doctors had resisted, the Kings took matters into their own hands.

Ashya had successful surgery to remove the brain tumor. Well done. Then, the doctors wanted to follow up with chemotherapy and X-ray radiation. Seeing other children who were turned into unresponsive vegetables by the recommended treatment motivated the Kings to find a better alternative.

The doctors for England's National Health Service (NHS) told the parents, and later the press, that proton therapy was no better than what they offered. They were either ignorant or deceitful — not a very favorable range of possibility.

In their disputes over treatment, the Kings presented the fruits of their research regarding alternatives to radiation and chemotherapy, pleading that proton therapy would be a better course of action. In response, one of the doctors reminded them that the NHS could get a legal order to take away custody of Ashya if the parents were uncooperative. It was that threat (later denied by the doctor) that led them to plot their escape to take Ashya surreptitiously out of England for treatment in Prague.

They prepared for every eventuality, getting a wheelchair, medications, food and equipment (including a battery charger for the feeding machine). Every day they took Ashya out of the hospital to get fresh air for an increasing length of time, ultimately reaching a couple of hours. In that way, when they had made their escape, their absence wasn't suspected right away. It's all very suspenseful to read.

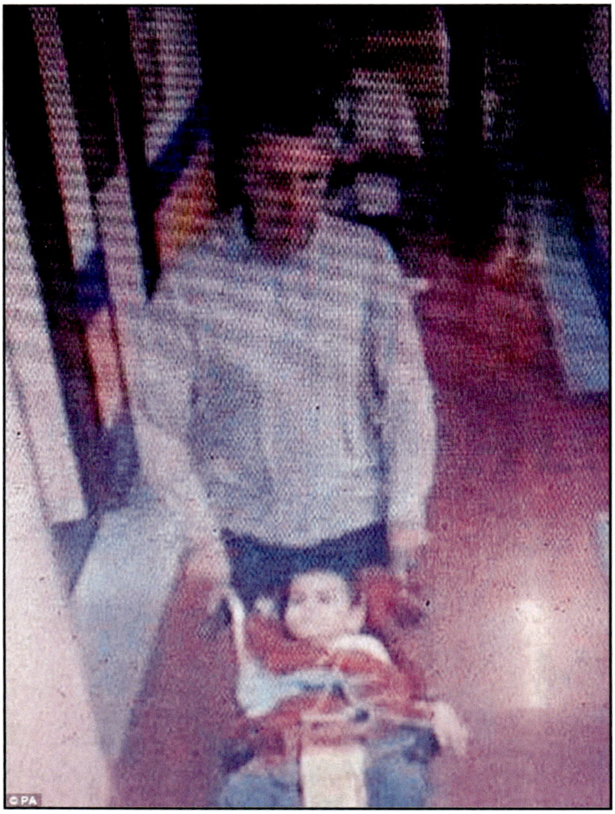

An actual frame from a security camera video of the Kings removing their son from the hospital. Trying to look normal, they were going crazy inside. They went right to the ferry terminal and were headed for France before their absence was detected.

The medical authorities had no idea the Kings were so well prepared. They assumed that on a whim they had just grabbed Ashya and taken him away. That wasn't the case, but not knowing that, the doctors feared Ashya's well-being was endangered. So they obtained an international arrest warrant for endangering the life and safety of a minor. Interpol got on the case and posted notices around Europe. Their flight made it onto the news worldwide.

The plan was for the Kings to reach their vacation home in Spain, and then find their way to Prague to the proton therapy center there, with whom they had been in close contact. After driving all night, they did reach Spain, but were spotted at a motel where the parents were arrested and jailed leaving their six other children to fend for themselves. Ashya was taken to a local hospital. One of their sons posted their plight on social media, with videos showing that Ashya was okay and explaining their intention to get the treatment that had been denied them. In the ensuing public response, more than 250,000 people signed petitions to free the parents. The King's Spanish attorney showed that the warrant was improper because the parents weren't endangering Ashya. Finally, the British government withdrew the warrant, the parents were freed, and Ashya made it to Prague, where he was treated successfully.

Any reasonable amount of research and observation would tell you Ashya's doctors were mistaken, defensive, and uninformed. Yet, from their own point of view, how would it work if every parent that found some new thrilling treatment wanted to remove their child from standard procedures? Further, they decried the false hope given to every child with a brain tumor whose parents would ask for proton therapy when it wasn't possible. The medical establishment was caught in a bind, for sure, to which their response was at the very least unfortunate, if not unethical. The doctors were bombarded with negative emails and letters, some of them threatening. The case stirred up a real hornets' nest of outrage.

The Kings knew that chemotherapy and radiation would not bring Ashya out of his partial paralysis. It would more than likely kill him. Who was actually risking Ashya's life? Can you get an arrest warrant for the doctors? Ultimately, the NHS got the last word, getting the public to turn on the Kings when they were told (falsely) that the parents' actions in refusing chemotherapy had reduced Ashya's chances of survival by 50%. The statistic was made up and demonstrably false. Fake news, we would say today. Yet, hey continued to repeat that false statistic.

Even the prime minister got involved. Eventually, the NHS paid for the proton therapy. Under public scrutiny, the doctors did some of the things they should have done up front, such as sending Ashya's MRIs to Prague. This story has a happy ending, sort of.

Here are some of the comments on the internet regarding the King case.

Hypocrites! The nasty egotistical doctors who fought against Ashya's right to live are all smiles and now admitting the treatment would work. They knew the treatment WOULD work but did not want to open the 'floodgates.' They now have to state that they will send other children with the same kind of cancer to countries where they administer Proton Therapy. They didn't want to spend NHS money on saving children's lives and still don't. How will the British public know if they actually will send ill children abroad for the treatment ? !

Well, well, well, the "authorities" now agree this treatment works and they are bringing it to the UK. So obviously it wasn't fully studied in the first place and just rejected out of hand by the same "authorities"! How many children in the meantime have died because these self same "authorities" didn't do their jobs properly, just made decisions without checking the evidence and without any thought for those that might have benefited from what is obviously an effective treatment. Seems another case of life being measured in ££££. "Sorry children, we don't want to have to pay for your treatment, you'll just have to die!"

I wrote the center in Prague and asked them about the King case. They said they received hundreds of emails every day from people inquiring about proton therapy, often for cases that didn't qualify. Their business increased for private pays, but the NHS stopped sending them patients. Here is a link to the British site for the Prague center: http://ukprotontherapy.co.uk/

Further down the road, the doctors and staff had their say in a documentary done by the BBC and a study done by local officials. The doctors continued to repeat the completely bogus statistic that by refusing chemotherapy, the Kings had reduced the survival rate for Ashya by half, not acknowledging that proton therapy had done the job. The doctors claimed that they had Ashya's best interests in mind and were thwarted by irrational parents who were religious zealots (Jehovah's Witnesses) whose actions threatened their son.

After the BBC program aired, social media then poured abuse onto the Kings who felt it was undeserved and that their story and motives weren't fairly presented. After the Kings returned to England, the health service refused to have anything more to do with them, causing them to leave and go back to Spain for appropriate physical and speech therapy. All this is very well documented on the internet. A search under "Ashya King" will bring up an abundance of material. The most recent result I could find was January of 2017. I presume that young Ashya continues to recover and regain his mobility and speech.

Here is a video of Ashya three years after his proton treatment: http://www.mirror.co.uk/news/uk-news/ashya-king-is-cancer-free-9813409.

Once on the offensive, the NHS then went on to issue a clear warning about the marketing of "emerging treatments," stating unequivocally that "some overseas clinics providing proton beam therapy heavily market their services to parents who are understandably desperate to get treatment for their children." The statement added that it's "not clear whether all children treated privately abroad are treated appropriately." I would ask, how clear is it that patients being treated in the United Kingdom are being treated appropriately?

I found this news article online:

Ashya King, the boy with a brain tumour whose parents disappeared with him to Spain because they did not want the kind of radiotherapy available in the UK, will have his treatment paid for by the NHS after all, it has been revealed. NHS England has agreed to fund proton beam therapy for Ashya under the reciprocal healthcare arrangements that exist within the EU, on the basis that the five-year-old needs a course of radiotherapy as a matter of urgency and, if he is to recover, he must have it now in Prague, where he has been taken by his family.

Ashya's case had previously been turned down by a specialist expert panel of doctors, on the basis that proton beam therapy offers no benefit that the child could not get from standard radiotherapy in the UK.

The specialist panel examines all the cases of children who might benefit from proton beam therapy brought to them by NHS hospitals and can make the decision to send them abroad – usually to the United States – for treatment.

The U-turn by NHS England, because of the application within the EU rules rather than normal NHS protocol, may make other parents who would prefer proton beam therapy to standard radiotherapy for their child seek to take them abroad.

In Ashya's case, however, doctors maintained that protons offered no advantage, because the entire brain and spine would have to be irradiated, whichever method was used. I'm sure those doctors who claimed that proton therapy had no advantage were the same "specialists" who would "reassure" the Kings about the treatment that awaited Ashya in Southampton. The experts' declarative statements are based on little knowledge or evidence. Even in the United States, where the insurance industry has put up a stiff fight against covering proton therapy, they have relented for pediatric cancers, especially brain tumors, for which protons are clearly superior, a position backed up by substantial clinical evidence.

Meanwhile, a spokesperson for University Hospital Southampton NHS Foundation Trust told MailOnline:

From the moment we performed life-saving surgery to remove Ashya's brain tumour, our interest was only ever in providing the best care and treatment for him. We cooperated fully with his parents and were in the process of arranging a safe transfer to the Proton Therapy Center in Prague at their request when he was removed from our hospital without warning. We have, and always will, dispute the King family's version of events.

How's that for revisionist history! They were arranging for proton therapy? And didn't tell the parents after all their pleas? The Kings took their entire journey for nothing? Hardly. What about the statement above that says the proton therapy was approved through a special EU provision and not through normal NHS procedures as they claimed. No wonder the Kings wrote this book to express their side of the story.

In March of 2018 a newspaper article in England gave an update on Ashya's cancer journey. The strain of the whole ordeal had led his parents to the verge of divorce, but then they reconciled. Here is their description of Ashya's current condition.

Now after the most recent MRI scans in Southampton show no signs of a tumour, Ashya is as close as possible to being given the all-clear.

The chatty eight-year old enjoys riding his bike and playing football like any other boy in his class, despite a slight weakness in his right side from the brain surgery in Southampton. . . . Dr Hernan Cortes Funes, head of oncology at the HC Marbella International hospital in Spain who has treated Ashya for three years, told the Daily Mail: "This isn't an exact science but three-and-a-half years is a good time to presume he won't relapse."

(For the entire article, see: https://www.telegraph.co.uk/news/2018/03/03/ashya-king-cleared-cancer-three-years-parents-abducted-hospital/).

A series of articles responded to the Kings' appearance on Good Morning Britain in March (2018). One such article reported Ashya King is now a happy little eight-year-old boy who aspires to be a chef. The family lives in Portsmouth, where Ashya loves to run and play soccer with his mates.

What strikes me is the normalcy he has reached, as opposed to the almost certain prognosis that the prescribed treatment in England would have left him a vegetable. This is clearly a huge, very visible triumph for Ashya King and his family. The hospital from which they fled continues to dispute the Kings' version of the events. Meanwhile, despite resistance from some quarters, proton therapy has been taking root in the United Kingdom with at least six centers planned and one that just opened.

Yet, although proton therapy will soon be available in the UK, the disinformation continues. Karol Sikora, the respected

Medical Director of CancerPartnersUK, said: "By the time they will be operational they will be obsolete." Another critic said, "What is most shocking is that many cancer victims may be denied treatment as so much is being invested in these white elephants." Not true of course. The technology does keep improving, as it should, but the older technology is not obsolete.

One doctor proclaimed: "These machines only work for a small number of cancer patients." He went on: "They will also cost some £50million ($67,600,000) a year to run. Last year 134 UK patients used this treatment. This is . . . economic madness."

The situation in the UK typifies, in some ways, the faulty attitudes and criticisms experienced here in the US, with seemingly respected experts calling proton therapy ridiculous or useless or unproven. Even while the NHS had been battling with the Kings, they were moving forward on building their own proton centers. In addition, a company called Proton-Partners International is developing five privately run proton centers in the UK, the first of which is now open (2018) in Newport, South Wales. Here is their news video: https://www.youtube.com/watch?v=knmJDG8seLQ. They are building other proton centers in Reading, Liverpool, Northampton, and London. I believe these will all have smaller equipment in single treatment rooms. All five, then, would have slightly less capacity than the two NHS centers.

CONCLUSION

The story of Ashya King in the book *Saving Ashya* by Naghmeh King could easily have been about any number of children (and adults) denied proton therapy by the medical establishment. Even while they were denying protons as unnecessary they were building their own centers to offer it. The promise of proton therapy is great news. Some day protons will be widely known and available, partly because of determined parents like the Kings.

SHARE AND REVIEW

Right now, my life's focus is on getting out the word about proton therapy. In almost every conversation in which I bring up the subject, the other parties are unaware of proton therapy. Further, they all tell stories about a friend or relative who had a very difficult time with their cancer treatment. If only they had known.

Even when someone tells me in great anguish that they have been diagnosed with cancer, my presentation of the potential of proton therapy often goes nowhere. They either forget it or dismiss it or mention it to their doctor who warns against it.

It's a sad state of affairs that we must all work so hard to get proton therapy, and then to have it covered by insurance. Now that you have read this book to the very end, I assume that you found this information useful. Please help to spread the word by telling others about this book (which also exists in ebook format). And, right now, while it is on your mind, go to Amazon.com and leave a positive review. If your response isn't positive, then please write me and express your opinion and suggestions directly (robert@ProtonTherapyBook.com). I want to get this right. You can help. Many thanks.

NOTES:

NOTES:

Made in the USA
Coppell, TX
09 February 2023

12552519R00083